Breathless to Live

Breathless to Live

by

Kenneth M. Hay
M.B.E., MA., M.D., F.R.C.G.P.

His Autobiography

The Pentland Press Limited
Edinburgh · Cambridge · Durham

First published in 1994 by
The Pentland Press Ltd.
1 Hutton Close
South Church
Bishop Auckland
Durham

ISBN 1 85821 165 4

Typeset by Elite Typesetting Techniques, Southampton.
Printed and bound by Antony Rowe Ltd., Chippenham.

In Memory of Ursula Beatrice Hay (Sue)

My beloved wife, companion and helpmate
for forty-six years

Contents

Foreword
by George Hearn, M.B.E., M.D., F.R.C.P.

It is a privilege to be invited to write a brief foreword to this excellent medical autobiography. It is of great interest to me, now well into my eighties, for in the last few years I have acquired the intuition to see, in 3D as it were, the lives of those whom I have known for many years, seeing them, not only as they are now, but in their becoming. This gives me much joy, to be able to recall in the failing octogenarian the vigour and the splendour of that active life in the making fifty or more years before.

This is what Michael Hay has done for us here, in this modest, unpretentious absorbing record of the tranquil family atmosphere of his privileged childhood, of the determination with which he overcame his asthma, to such good effect that it was years after we first worked together that I learned that he was troubled in this way, to the serious disturbance of his years of education, of his medical studies at Bart's, and of the whole of his medical life, spread out for us from its beginning to its end, to the point that now, in his retirement, he has the leisure to recall it in all its interest and compassion.

As he records, we first met in 1947 when he came to Dudley Road Hospital, Birmingham, performing the duties of house physician, but carrying the status of Grade Three Registrar, a training or refresher category created for those returning to civil hospital life after years in the Forces where they had exercised their own independent clinical judgement. And this he continued to do, a first class doctor who gave us so much help as we dealt with the large number of sick people who flooded into the hospital at that time from the battered city of Birmingham. I was one of the recently appointed physicians, having spent the previous six years in the R.A.M.C. He and I have remained good friends since, not seeing one another frequently, but when we did meet, taking up where we left off, both developing, both older, both with greater experience.

As I read these pages, I was reminded of Winston Churchill's memorable comment which has remained in my mind these fifty years: 'Men fell from the air in flames, or were smothered, often slowly, in the dark recesses of the sea . . . and withal, as an individual, he preserved through these torments the glories of a reasonable and compassionate mind.' (1) This book reveals how this particular 'reasonable and compassionate mind' reacted with this terrible Twentieth Century, by responding to the needs of his fellows wherever he happened to be, giving them hope and reaching out to them in friendship.

The enquiring mind was active, too. His serendipidous involvement with the mysteries of dark adapted vision in the R.A.F. led, on his return to civil life, to his fascinated exploration of migraine, in which field he acquired a more than local reputation, and a clinical and scientific interest which illuminated his mind and his practice.

We can be grateful that he has given us this book, which can be commended without reserve. Perhaps a friend may be allowed to express admiration, tinged with regret, for the skill with which he hides from his readers any reference to a private life which those of us who have been privileged from time to time to observe from without have seen as much blessed.

(1) Winston S. Churchill (1942) *The World Crisis 1911–1918*,
                                    Macmillan, London, p20.

Chapter 1

Asthma

Thomas Willis (1621-1675) writing about asthma made the following observations. 'Among the diseases whereby the region of the breath is wont to be infested, if you regard their tyranny and cruelty, an asthma doth not deserve the last place: for there is scarce anything more sharp and terrible than the fits thereof: the organs of breathing and the precordia themselves, which are the foundations and pillars of life, are shaken by the disease as by an earthquake, and so totter that nothing less than the ruins of the whole animal fabrick seems to be threatened: for breathing, whereby we chiefly live is very much hindered by the assault of this disease, and is in danger or runs the risque of being quite taken away.'

I have been subject to asthma from an early age, and have had to rely on such medicaments as were available at different times to keep it sufficiently under control to enable me to lead a fairly normal life. Before the age when I started to go to school it was possible to accept this like other disabilities which afflict some people as part of the natural order of things provided one is lucky, as I was, in getting good family support and care. It is later on in the school years that the difficulties became more serious when it is realized that one is different to the majority of the class and unable to compete effectively in the more strenuous games. Once these problems had been weathered and I had become more mature it became easier to adapt to life and with guile, dissimulation, and the sensible use of modern medicaments to get by without being looked upon as being abnormal and deserving of condescension.

Asthma is no new disorder, and references were made to it in the Hippocratic writings of 400 BC. Aretaeus (c. AD 200) gives a good description of it. He writes 'If from running, gymnastic exercises or any other work the breathing become difficult it is called asthma, and the disease orthopnoea is also called asthma, for in the paroxysms the patients also pant for breath. The disease is called orthopnoea because it is only in the erect position that they breathe freely, for when reclined there is a sense of suffocation . . .'

Between attacks the asthmatic appears to be normal, but can become breathless on exertion, after heavy meals and in conditions of fog and cold. There are many other factors which can help to precipitate attacks such as allergy, infections, and stress leading to fatigue. Together with the disabilities caused by asthma there can be profound feelings of inferiority and failure especially in adolescence. Nowadays a better scientific understanding of the condition has led to better forms of treatment together with a more sympathetic knowledge of the psychological needs of patients, and the prospects for asthmatics are vastly improved.

Boys, in middle class families, before the last war were often sent away to preparatory boarding schools at the age of seven and, later on, having taken an examination called the Common Entrance they went to one of the great traditional public schools to be made ready for the universities, the armed services, or the church. By these means they met the 'right people' and learned their place in the social order and what was expected of a gentleman in manners, speech, and prejudices. Though much of the education left one a sound and worthy citizen if one came through unscathed, it also meant that one had a limited outlook and experience of the problems of the day.

I failed to survive the rigours of both my preparatory and my public school as my asthma got out of control. Before going to my preparatory school I had been a day boy at Mr Gibbs' in Sloane Street in London taking myself there by bus which in those days was often open to the elements on top, which is where I and other boys would choose to sit if possible. We wore bright-red school caps and were taught the fundamentals of the three R's by a kindly staff. I enjoyed that school and the special lectures on natural history, and the games and events provided for us by Mr Gibbs.

Such asthma attacks as I used to get then usually occurred at night or when London was shrouded in one of its winter pea-soup fogs. Then I would sit up in bed inhaling Potter's Asthma Cure or a similar preparation called Nimrod. A match would be applied to a little cone of the powder which would then sparkle away releasing clouds of smoke containing the ingredients to stop the attacks. Sometimes our G.P. would be summoned; in our case a Dr Attlee who was always smartly dressed and groomed and who inspired a feeling of confidence and reassurance though I disliked his medicines containing iodine and stramonium among other ingredients. If these were not enough, adrenaline would be given by injection or ephedrine administered by mouth. Both would make my heart beat faster and give feelings of restlessness and unease, though the relief from breathing difficulties was marvellous.

It was at about this time in my life that I first realised that asthma could be a disabling handicap. The event itself was trivial, but left me feeling inadequate and a failure. In the summer we went on family holidays to the seaside and this time it was in North Wales at Fairbourne. Lodgings were taken in a house with a landlady and packing-cases of food were sent in advance from the Army and Navy Stores in London. Nanny came with us and joined in the picnics and the joys of messing about after shrimps and prawns which were brought back to be boiled and then eaten with relish. There was sea bathing. There were sands and rock pools to be explored with the exciting backdrop of the Welsh mountains.

My father would join us at weekends, though he never really liked family holidays in lodgings preferring to go salmon and trout fishing in Scotland for his annual recreation. Possibly, with ideas of following in his footsteps, I thought it would be a good idea to fish for bigger game than shrimps and prawns.

There is a railway bridge over the Mawddach estuary with a footpath beside it. From this it was possible to dangle a wire contraption armed with several hooks called a paternoster. This was baited with lugworms dug up from the sands. Nanny, as usual, was with us to keep an eye on our activities and to relish our excitement. However, the sport was slow, most of the bait being taken by small inedible shore crabs; but the occasional dab was hauled in. As always, one was reluctant to leave lest one missed the monster just waiting to be caught; so time passed and the evening train to take us back to our lodgings and tea hove in sight. The sun was shining, we had caught some fish and all was well, except that we had to run to catch the train. Inevitably this brought on a fit of wheezing and slowed me up.

Then it was that a tall man with a greying, clipped moustache, rubicund complexion, and the loud, harsh voice of military authority decided to join in the fun. Waving his arms in a sort of mock choleric semaphore he shouted at me 'Run, boy, run, or you will be late for your funeral'. There was nothing kindly in his hectoring and I felt deeply humiliated and frightened. For the first time it really came home to me that there was something wrong with me; that in some ways I was different to others; that I was physically unable to do what was expected of me, and that I might be a failure.

That night I had a particularly bad attack of asthma and my poor mother had to administer medicines and Potter's Asthma Cure while trying to cheer me up by singing my favourite songs to me, including always Jerusalem and John Brown's Body. My health was a great anxiety to her, but she never let me see this and was always at hand to help and reassure.

My immediate family, Nanny, and my godmother Aunt Kit, a sister of my mother, were my unfailing support through childhood, and without them I would never have succeeded in living a more or less normal and enjoyable life.

Later on in school days there were to be others on whom I came to rely, notably Verney and Phyllis Kitchin to whose tutorial establishment I was to be sent after my health had broken down at boarding school. They lived at Château D'Oex in Switzerland, and the clean air and altitude of the Alps were thought to be beneficial to those with chest complaints; and there was to prove some justification for this idea in my case.

Nowadays a lot is known about the factors causing asthma, and a great deal of research is being done in many countries, while the pharmaceutical industry is coming up with a host of new remedies which were not available before the last war. It was, then, always a temptation to the medical profession to fall back on the notion of a 'functional disorder' without defining or understanding what they meant by the term. Usually a weakness of will was implied with the threat of the prospect of a life of limited opportunities. But, as so often happens in medicine, clinical observation pre-dates scientific discovery. In 1552 Archbishop Hamilton, Primate of Scotland, sought the help of a certain physician Jerome Cardan of Milan, who advised him to give up sleeping on feather pillows and to take time off from business and studies.

This advice apparently met with success and now, in the twentieth century, we understand the rôles of allergic sensitivity to many kinds of irritants including household dusts, feathers, and animal hairs. Otherwise asthmatics, like victims of other forms of bad health, had to put up with the added horrors of bleeding, purging and cupping; in fact I was once dry cupped by a village doctor in Switzerland called in to see me for a bad attack of bronchitis. Vacuums were made in little flasks by warming the air within them with a taper and clapping them on my chest. As the air cooled a semi-vacuum was created which drew my flesh up painfully into the flask rendering me temporarily immobile.

My real problems were to come at boarding school where physical disabilities were a greater disadvantage to me than they had ever been before, living as one did in a close community where physical fitness and prowess were at a premium. It is a common practice nowadays to denigrate one's preparatory and public schools, but I remember the headmaster and staff of Highfield school as being on the whole friendly and kindly. My problem was getting whooping cough and measles on top of one another while there, and this set me back when I was on the road to recovery.

There was much about the school which I remember with pleasure. For instance, when I was 'off games' I would be allowed to walk along footpaths through the woods and heaths around the school. On one such occasion I got a glimpse of a golden oriole in all the splendour of his breeding summer plumage. Besides the bird life there were fascinating moths and insects to be found; I often collected the latter alive and transferred them to my desk to show to my friends, until the form master, raising the top of my desk, discovered them among exercise books and Latin grammars.

I also spent many afternoons in the well equipped library where there were some illustrated volumes about the First World War. They began to bring home to me something of the ordeals faced by my parents' generation and to realise what the men marching in the victory parade which I had seen, but been too young to understand, had survived. I began to ask myself why the numerous ex-service bands begging for money in the streets of London had not been treated as the heroes I now regarded them as.

The war had been won, and the world maps we studied in class were full of lands coloured in red to show that they were all part of the Great British Empire. However, there was growing instability on the home front leading up to the General Strike. Hyde Park was closed and full of army lorries to be used to maintain food supplies. My parents unable to get me back to school by train hired a private car to take me and another boy back to Highfield. Before we got out of London we came to a standstill presumably due to a road block or demonstration, and were ushered into a transport depot with the roller blind doors shut to await the passing of whatever trouble had developed.

The school chapel was a haven of peace where one could be alone with one's thoughts away from the hurly-burly of communal life, particularly so when the lights were dimmed for the Evensong sermon. My most unpleasant experience was being put into quarantine for supposed mumps when in reality I had a salivary gland stone which was painful especially on eating. I was alone with only the distant sounds of ordinary life; a taste of solitary confinement.

However, I was not making much headway academically or as regards my health, and my parents decided to get further advice, part of which was that I should go to school in Switzerland.

Not having been abroad, I was somewhat alarmed at the prospect of being so far from home. Various suggestions were made and a tutor with his wife came to tea with my parents to discuss this idea of my going to their tutorial establishment in the Alps. After tea I was introduced to them. They gushed with jollity and heartiness which left me feeling shy and awkward. Then I was asked about my interests. These included collecting butterflies and moths: and when I said this the comment bounced out 'oh, how interesting, you see my husband is a bugger too'. My father choked back a laugh into his handkerchief and my mother changed the subject leaving me mystified and apprehensive.

However, my luck was to change for the better. The next prospective tutor I was introduced to was Mr Vernon Kitchin who came to tea at our house in Hill Street with his wife Phyllis. Obviously, they were sincere and caring people, intelligent and interesting with a good sense of humour. It was arranged that I should spend some of the summer holidays at the Hôtel du Torrent in Château D'Oex with my parents to see how the Alps suited me.

I was thrilled by the mountains and the scenery. Everything seemed to be clean and unhurried, the people pleasant and cheerful. There was the soothing background sound of the mountain stream by the hotel interspersed with distant cowbells from the mountain pastures. I soon felt better in my health as I started to explore the paths up the valleys into the mountain foothills. There was quite a big English colony in Château D'Oex, some of the members of it having been interned there in prisoner exchanges in the First World War: there was an English preparatory school and an Anglican Church with its own English incumbent.

When the time approached for my father to leave me in the care of Mr and Mrs Kitchin at the Châlet du Vallon, I had lost most of my apprehensions. I had got to know many of the English ex-patriates some of whom were amusingly eccentric.

One was an elderly retired clergyman living at the Hôtel du Torrent called the Revd. Horace Hopkins. He was very much an evangelical and wore the dark frock coat and the sort of squashed bowler hat popular in Victorian times. His great joy in life was his collection of canaries. Once they escaped to his great distress and agitation. They were well fed birds and did not stray far in their freedom. An exciting hunt ensued, with me wielding a butterfly net and the hotel proprietor and his wife trying to shoo them back to their cages. I caught most of them in my butterfly net. For thanks, I was asked to tea in his rooms and given a signed and annotated copy of a book of *St. Paul's Letter to the Romans.*

The Châlet du Vallon was – and is – a traditional wooden brown-stained building typical of so many in Canton Vaud. At the back there was a long balcony looking out over meadows to a background of mountains dominated by a tall rocky peak called the Gumfluh. This was to become a familiar outdoor classroom where we were taught English, French, and Latin by Mr Kitchin, usually known as Verney. When the sun shone he would be stripped to the waist, though this exposure was not enough for him and the pants came off too during his siesta after lunch, when we were banned from the balcony, though children with their natural curiosity would peer down from the upstairs bedroom windows causing furious indignation. There was a young lady teacher called Miss Sadd, inevitably known as Jolly Sadd, and a French Mademoiselle.

The pupils were of both sexes and ranged in age from about nine to seventeen years of age. They were there for a variety of reasons mostly connected with ill health, and had been unable to thrive in the traditional school system.

Mr Kitchin was a scholarly man with a great love of English literature, and I can well remember his reading of Dickens and Kipling among other classics. He had an actor's ability to make the characters speak in well defined accents in the dialogues so that the personalities became real. This was particularly so in his reading of Blackmore's *Lorna Doone*. He was of medium height and physically strong: everything he did was done with enthusiasm which was catching, whether it was pursuing rare butterflies high in trees, or skating, or playing billiards with us. He honestly believed in the existence of fairies – the traditional kind – and showed us pictures of them said to have been photographed by Conan Doyle. He tended to be a shy man outside his circle of friends.

His wife, Phyllis, was more of an extrovert, a motherly person with a ready sense of humour. She would come round our bedrooms at night before she retired herself to see that all was well with us, and if we were awake though pretending to be asleep we would hear her repeating over our beds 'every day and in every way he is getting better and better' as she was a disciple of Professor Coue.

My health improved and I thoroughly enjoyed walks into the mountains and the expeditions laid on for us by the Kitchins. I had riding lessons from a Mr Massey who had been a cavalry-man in the war and had been shot in the chest: he had arrived in Château D'Oex under some scheme to release wounded P.O.W.s to neutral countries.

The local postman used to come in to teach us Swiss wood-carving and tell us stories and gossip; his fingers and thumbs were criss-crossed with scars from accidental cuts from his razor sharp tools. I also had piano lessons though the teacher was hardly an inspired one and I made little progress. But life was very pleasant and I lost much of my apprehensiveness. By this time I was about twelve years of age and facing the school common entrance examination prior to going to my father's old public school, Sherborne in Dorset.

A new French Mademoiselle had arrived to teach us to speak and read in her language. She despised us younger ones while favouring the older boys, and indulging in minor pranks with them. Plastic turds were left around and bags placed under cushions to make fart noises when the seat was sat on. It was her teasing that I most resented, and I planned some sort of prank in revenge, thought I have forgotten what it was now. However, I was reported to Mr Kitchin who, not knowing the truth of the unpleasantness, gave me an angry dressing down and a warning that I would have to leave unless I apologised.

This was all a bit of a storm in a teacup and eventually it was the Mademoiselle who had to go on grounds which, with my rather strict upbringing, I could only sense and not fully understand. At any rate I was deeply unhappy as I had come to love and depend on the Kitchins as people who had rescued me from feeling a failure to myself and family. In this disturbed and depressed state of mind I went up into the meadows footing a small mountain I had come to know well and lay down in the grass to think.

I drowsed off eventually and came to later in a relaxed and dreamy state. The world seemed to be a different place; the grass, the flowers, the warmth of the sun took on a unity which seemed timeless and devoid of all the niggles and worries of ordinary life. I lay there intensely happy, relaxed, and grateful to be part of so wonderful an experience inexpressible in words. All fears had disappeared and I knew that I had had a rare glimpse of a reality more certain than anything else in life. I returned happy and confident that I would cope with human problems which bewildered me.

This type of experience we know now to be quite common and they have been described by William James in *Varieties of Religious Experience*, by Sir Alistair Hardy, and they have been investigated by David Hay in his book *Exploring Inner Space*. Arthur Koestler describes a rather similar sort of feeling which he called the Oceanic Experience at a time when his life was in danger in the Spanish Civil War. Whatever its nature it is something I am glad to have had at that time and on a few occasions subsequently. There seems to be a wide sense of awareness quite the opposite of the narrow states of excitement generated by some group rituals and meetings where emotions are narrowly pitched and manipulated. There is some inconclusive evidence that brain states reflected in alpha rhythms are necessary at the times of such occurrences.

We had a lot of freedom and Verney – as we called him among ourselves – would show us on maps where to go and what to look out for in the way of scenery and natural history. Trips were organised to Gruyère, Gstaad, Gsteig, and to the Diablarets mountains. Sometimes we would camp out, sleeping in the hay barns of friendly farmers.

On one walk with a friend in the early spring we saw across the valley a spectacular avalanche with its sudden roar and a great cloud of snow scattered into the air around it. This was an added bonus to a memorable day when we had watched the attractive little alpine marmots emerging from their winter hibernation where the snow line had receded.

I must have given my parents a vivid description of the day, as my mother wrote back urgently warning me not to get too near avalanches. Although we had been quite safe in the shelter of a summer farm we were told by the Kitchins to say more precisely where we intended to go when on future walks into the mountains. There was skating and skiing in the winter and tennis in the summer.

However, all good things must come to an end! With the Common Entrance behind me and being fitter mentally and physically I was considered able to face the next stage of life at Sherborne School. I had come to love Verney and Phyllis Kitchin, their Châlet du Vallon, Château D'Oex and the Alps with its friendly people.

My gratitude to them has remained fresh throughout my life; small incidents, games, jokes, and fun come back to me easily like Verney inventing new and apt spoonerisms in the tradition of 'Kinquering congs their titles take' spoken by the originator of the genre the Revd Dr Spooner. As things were to turn out later on I would be returning to their care in a year or two following a breakdown in my health at Sherborne school.

Chapter 2

Childhood and Family

It can be a difficult and sometimes frightening task to write about one's own memories and experiences, and to look again at old photographs taken from early boyhood onwards. There are also old letters written to my parents from school: there is even one from my uncle Geoffrey congratulating my parents on my birth. This was written from the Western Front in World War One a few days before he was killed. From photographs of him and what I was told later he was a handsome, dashing and popular man. The admonishment given by the Pythoness at Delphi 'to learn to know thyself' and echoed by various sages subsequently, requires resolution if some of the traps of self deception are to be avoided.

My mother was in to her thirties when I was born, and she had waited five years before conception; this only came after consultations with one of the pioneer lady gynaecologists. I was not a robust infant, and later on developed bronchial asthma which has plagued me all my life. Now, thanks to better medical understanding and the advent of new medicaments, it has become much easier to control.

One of the main purposes of my writing is to show that it is now possible to have a full, enjoyable and, hopefully, useful life with this particular handicap, even if much of my boyhood was difficult and unpleasant on this account. However, it was my good fortune to have the affection, acceptance and support of people I have loved and admired, and without them there would only have been the perils of rejection and failure. Most middle class professional families expected much of their sons, especially if they were the only sons. Education at preparatory and public boarding schools was physically, if not mentally, demanding and weaknesses were not condoned.

The biggest lottery in life is to whom one was destined to be born and to have as parents, and also where and when one first saw the light of day.

My birth was in January 1915 at a time when 'the war to end all wars' was settling down to four years of massacre in the mud of Flanders, shattering for ever the earlier hopes of a short, brief campaign to be fought with enthusiasm in the cause of freedom, while England was safe from the threats of invasion as an island defended by a navy unbeatable since Nelson's days.

Air raids by Zeppelins and Gotha aircraft were soon to come, and my earliest memory was of being hustled in my pram by Nanny out of Kensington Gardens. Bombs had been dropped and I suppose that like the young of many animals I was sensitive to the general alarm and excitement without having any inkling of what it was all about. We were fleeing to the safety of our home in Vicarage Gardens off Kensington High Street, though later we were to move from there to St. Albans after some windows had been shattered in a later raid.

My first home where I was born was in St. James's Place in an old house now owned by the Royal Ocean Racing Club. My father ran a private medical practice from this house, which was reputed to be haunted by a ghost. It was at the end of a quiet cul-de-sac: quiet enough on one occasion for two waiters of Italian origin to go there to settle their feud with knives. My father, a reticent and peace loving man as a rule, could show resolution when occasion demanded it and after striding angrily from the house he seized the combatants by the scruffs of their necks while my terrified mother rang for the police.

Soon after the war started my father became a surgeon at the First London General Hospital, a wartime branch of St. Bartholomew's dedicated to the care of the war wounded from the Western Front. My father was a doctor, essentially a general practitioner, but he soon found he had a flair for surgery which was helped by his being ambidextrous. The workload increased as the war progressed, and included plastic surgery, then being developed by Sir Harold Gillies. Many of the wounds were heavily infected especially so when the victims had lain out in no-man's-land, sometimes for days, before being rescued: antibiotics had not then been invented.

He was a tall, handsome man with a long face which had earned him the nickname of horsey at school. His father, my grandfather, was a wealthy and successful City of London merchant, though he had died before I was born. His wife, my grandmother, came from an aristocratic family of the Victorian vintage. All the time I knew her she was dressed in widow's deepest black modelling herself in this as in other ways on Queen Victoria.

There were four sons, Alan the eldest who inherited the family business, John who was a brilliant engineer and inventor, but who came to be regarded as the family skeleton in the cupboard due to his liaison with a chorus girl who eventually became his wife and who looked after him in his final illness when he was found to have T.B. Then came my father Kenneth: lastly there was poor Geoffrey killed in the first year of the war.

Of the girls there was Mary who married a Scots business man. I found her to be a forthright and formidable aunt with an upper lip which reminded me of the face of the turtles I had seen in the London zoo. Then came Aunt Bea – short for Beatrice – also a formidable character in the eyes of young children.

Aunt Connie was married to a Yorkshire steel merchant, but became badly afflicted with Parkinsonism. Despite this handicap she liked to follow the local hunt, literally up hill and down dale, in a pony trap with the reins tied round her wrists. Excitement of the chase and poor control meant that Connie with the pony and trap would sometimes end in a ditch. A devoted chauffeur/groom following in a car would come to the rescue and sort things out. She also liked to go to the theatre, and this meant a lot of effort and planning by my parents to manoeuvre her large frame and wheelchair into a carefully selected place in the auditorium.

Lastly, there was Aunt Cis who devoted her life to music and to running the family farm. I remember her as a large active lady usually dressed in severely cut tweeds with a pork pie hat complete with feather on her head when she took us out in the dog-cart. Everything was correct, the pony and trap having been immaculately polished by the efficient groom and stable lad. The hairy horse-rug over my aunt's knees, the whip held at the correct angle and the steady movements of the pony's rump made these expeditions memorable, and so much more stylish a form of travel than we enjoy today in cars.

In the best sense of the term, my father had been a bit of a family rebel. Medicine was not considered to be of high enough class, and the local doctor when he did a professional call was not admitted through the front door, but was let in through a lesser side one. However, my father studied medicine at Cambridge University where he rowed in his college eight, and later at St. Bartholomew's Hospital in the City of London. He did well, and after qualification became house physician to Sir Dyce Duckworth one of the medical consultants. It is recorded that once, while a resident in the hospital, he invited his mother to tea in his rooms: when it came to pouring out from the teapot two cockroaches appeared from the spout causing horror and consternation to my disconcerted Granny.

Later, he went to work at a hospital at Shadwell in a poor area where he got experience of a very different and rougher society than the one in which he had been brought up. There was no N.H.S. then, but doctors and nurses were respected so that they would safely move in areas where policemen had to go in pairs. My father and the other doctors habitually wore, as part of their uniforms, gold watches and chains, and when one was stolen, the hospital let it be known that no more patients would be treated from the area where the theft occurred until it was returned, which it was within a few hours. This sort of rough justice was generally understood and accepted.

My father often talked about his days there, and he retained an interest in the area until late in his life, as he did voluntary medical work for a children's crèche, to which we were expected to contribute redundant toys and clothes. He was interested in the medical aspects of working conditions and was an early member of the Industrial Welfare Society which gave the impetus to much of what is now known as the discipline of industrial medicine. Fond as he was of his family home of Sacombe in Hertfordshire and the country surrounding it, his true love was London and its clubs and institutions like the Royal Society of Medicine, and the Royal Institution of which he was made a 'visitor'. He was an avid reader of books, usually of biography, travel or the classics as he understood Greek and Latin. By nature kindly, possibly too unassertive, he was called upon to help settle rows among members of his family which he did with tolerance and commonsense.

I owe him a great debt of gratitude for all the support he gave me during my childhood and adolescence when I was in danger of being disabled by asthma and prevented from pursuing a medical or other acceptable career.

My mother was the daughter of a City of London wine merchant who lived in a small village near Ware in Hertfordshire. He came of Quaker stock and on marriage to my maternal grandmother, who was a Roman Catholic, both agreed to become members of the Church of England. I remember him as a kindly patriarchal figure with a white beard which I greatly admired. He was always welcoming and ready to entertain children, and we missed him greatly when he died soon after he retired when he had entered his eighties. My maternal grandmother was a lively talented and spontaneous person, but she died from typhoid fever while I was yet a baby. They had five daughters and no sons: there was Katherine known by all as Aunt Kit, Rachel my mother, Dodo, Barbara and Chris.

My mother was a fine cellist and musician and enjoyed to the full the musical life of London. She had a romantic nature and expectations for the success and good futures for her children which were perhaps set too high for our comfort. She had a kindly nature and did charitable work among young girls who had landed in welfare homes after their own families had failed them. In consequence, we had a number of these girls engaged as domestics. My mother trained them in their work, and they kept up with her in later years after they had married and started families. In fact some of them with their husbands came to her memorial service which was a tribute to my mother for the help she gave them.

When I was a few weeks old and was living in the family home in St. James's Place, Miss Amy Thompson came to be my Nanny and to help my mother in the house. She was then a young girl of twenty-two. She became my mother's friend and confidante in the war years and remained with us until my sisters and I were too old to need a nanny, leaving to help other families, including an Anglo-American one in the United States. Her charges became her lifelong friends and still keep in touch with her.

She is now ninety-nine years old, but retains a lively mind and memory as she delights in talking of old times with humour and insight into the foibles of some of the more eccentric friends and members of my family. Of slight build with good clear cut features she must have been very attractive as a young girl. I knew the story of how, pushing me out in my pram to get the air of St. James's Park, the Prince of Wales in khaki uniform peeped round the hood of the pram to admire the baby, doubtless as an excuse to have a chat with an attractive young nanny. It is only recently that she told me that they met more than once when I was being given an airing in the pram. In those days it seems that security measures for members of the Royal Family did not have to be as tight as they are now.

She never married despite her fondness for children and her ready enjoyment of life. It has been rumoured that a boy friend had been killed in France, and she spent some years of her retirement looking after a brother who had been badly injured at the front.

Totally unselfish and loyal, with a ready sense of humour to soften a brisk common sense efficiency, she belongs to a breed which is all too rare in the modern world. She loved to take us as children to the annual fun-fairs at Olympia, which was an added attraction to the Mills' family circus which was held in the Christmas holidays. She was always ready to take us out by train or coach to places like Brighton, and I remember well my first trip in a speed-boat at that resort.

On family seaside holidays she put up with our shrimp and prawn catching and went with us on fishing trips with the local boatmen. She kept us tidy and clean, telling off my sister Anne who had accepted an invitation from a friendly keeper at the London Zoo to sit on the back of an amiable but wet hippopotamus and so soil her Sunday clothes.

My father was a Fellow of the Zoo and had privileges on Sundays when the general public were excluded. I, too, got a telling off for having candle grease on my blue serge suit after going to a children's service and had graciously been allowed to join a procession up the aisle carrying a lighted candle.

The whole family owe our Nanny a tremendous debt of gratitude for all her friendship, good humour and selfless help to us over a great many years. We visit her in her home and speak to her regularly on the telephone. She loves to look through old family photograph albums, and once while doing this she found a picture of her own mother which I had taken at the age of seven. I had had my tonsils out and had been sent to recuperate in Bournemouth where her mother lived. I had been given a Box Brownie camera as compensation for the operation and had been trying it out. This picture made Nanny recall, among other things, that her mother as a child had seen the veterans of the Crimea war returning.

She used to take us as children to see many of the Royal occasions and the parades such as the Changing of the Guard at Buckingham Palace. The hush of expectancy followed by an increasing crescendo of cheering from the crowds, and then the resplendent state coaches, Life Guards on their horses and the flag waving all made a deep impression on us.

During the First World War Nanny moved with the family to a small house in Vicarage Garden, and later to St. Albans. After

the war she came with us to Hill Street which was my home
during the rest of my childhood. Her loyalty and unselfishness
we took for granted and she shared our joys and sorrows. Even
after her retirement we have turned to her at times of family
illness, and she helped my wife and myself to look after our
children when my wife had to go into hospital for a major
operation.

As the years go by I realise more clearly than ever what a
debt of gratitude my family owe her.

The long days with a small baby were lonely times for my
mother with my father away at his hospital and the bad news
from the front did not allay the anxieties and fears of her
sensitive nature. It was under these circumstances that she saw
the ghost of St. James's Place. Young servants had, from time to
time, complained that the house was haunted, but their fears
had been dismissed as being fanciful.

One day my mother was getting ready to go out to the shops
and was struggling into her overcoat in a front room of the
house and seeing a servant, as she thought, gazing out of the
window asked to be helped on with her coat. At this the figure
vanished leaving my mother bewildered and fearful that she
was going mad. She got the opinion of a distinguished neurologist, Sir Henry Head, to whom she was distantly related. He
made the diagnosis of a potentially fatal brain disease. But,
remembering the fears of servants about the place being
haunted, my mother went to a local library and found the story
of the lady supposed to have been murdered in that house.

Over the years I have heard one or two first hand accounts of
rather similar apparitions being seen, usually when anxiety and
fatigue was being experienced by the tellers of these tales. As
told to me these experiences were more strange than alarming,
and perhaps some sort of eidetic imagery is responsible for
them.

Eventually the war ended with the Armistice and we moved
to a large, tall house in Hill Street in London's Mayfair. It was
joined to the houses either side of it: there were a hundred
stairs from the ground floor to the top storey, and there was a

further flight of stairs leading to the basement and kitchen quarters. It was spacious, inconvenient to run, and without any garden or access to the outside world other than the front or kitchen doors; there was also the drawing room balcony which overlooked the street. From this observation point we children would watch the comings and goings of people from above.

There were the gas-lamp lighters with their burning torches at the end of long poles, muffin men shouting their wares, and street bands usually of ex-service men then on a pitiful dole and unemployed after demobilization. One of our favourites was the barrel organ lady, a cheery gap-toothed old woman, her black dress covered by a colourful shawl and a scarf round her head. She would exchange greetings with us as we threw pennies to her from the balcony.

There was no central heating then, and every room had coal fires. The coal came up from the basement by a lift which worked on a system of ropes and wheels. It took a good deal of heaving to bring it up to the top floors and it was very noisy. Coal fires meant chimney sweeps had to come at regular intervals and this needed that everything had to be draped in sheets to catch the soot which evaded the sweeper's bag.

Coal fires being the normal method of house heating meant that in still, damp weather conditions in winter we would suffer the famous London pea-souper fogs which had particularly nasty or even dangerous effects on those with breathing disorders. They also left a great deal of grime about on paintwork and furniture. To escape them we would go for long stays with Granny Hay at Sacombe in the Hertfordshire countryside where there was a nursery suite and where for most of the time we lived apart from the life of the rest of the house.

Sacombe was a wonderful experience in more ways than one. The journey by train from Liverpool Street station to Ware took us through some of the grimier parts of London with endless terrace houses and small backyards with the family washing set out on clothes lines. The people living there seemed to us to be almost of a different race in their cramped surroundings after our more spacious ones.

At Ware station we would be met by Mr Longland the chauffeur in a Fiat limousine, a noisy but roomy machine. I would sit in the passenger seat next to Mr Longland who would regale me with all the local gossip. The road eventually arrived at a turning to a private farm track through farmland and meadows. At various points there were cattle gates to be opened and cottages housing familiar faces. As we got nearer to the house, fears and apprehensions would grow about how we would be received and what would be the inevitable criticisms about our appearances or behaviour – 'children should be seen and not heard' – was an aphorism from these days which remains in my memory.

We would arrive eventually at the imposing portico of Sacombe House in its setting of Sacombe Park. A bell pull would be pulled and after a wait of what could seem to us to be long minutes the great mahogany doors would be opened by Williams the butler. Then one of our formidable aunts would greet us in the large front hall in which there were marble busts in the Roman classical tradition.

Then, with growing feelings of apprehension, we would pass into the magnificent central hall with a short, central staircase leading to a landing on each side of which a further flight of stairs would lead to a sort of gallery off which were the bedrooms and Aunt Bea's private office. The hall itself extended to the top of the building where there was a large dome shaped sky-light.

The nursery quarters, where we were destined to stay, were large and comfortable but set back near the servants' wing. In all likelihood we would have been told 'not to make any noise because Granny was resting', so we were glad to arrive in the more homely nursery suite away from the grander parts of the house. Later, after tea, we would be scrubbed and dressed in clean best clothes to greet Granny in her drawing room. This was a bit of an ordeal when we were quite young and we were known to embarrass our Nanny by having a paddy outside the door. When we entered we found Granny, a little old lady dressed in black, her hair parted in the middle and swept severely back to a bun. She would be seated in an armchair by the fire with her black-booted feet on a tuffet. Her wrinkled old face would show no emotion as we approached to give the ritual kisses, one on each parchment cheek and say 'good evening'. 'Good evening who?' would come the answer, and then we would say correctly 'good evening, Granny'. After that we might be given a story or asked to learn a poem.

Looking back I can see that in some ways she was a lonely widow missing an active and popular husband. She made it her role to maintain a way of life which had been shattered by the First World War. Her model was the pre-war landed aristocracy and this way of life had needed the injection of wealth from a city business for its maintenance. This my grandfather and my Uncle Alan were able to provide through a family firm dealing in non-ferrous metals and, at one time, shipping. Granny ruled her family and her domestic staff with firmness and decision and was generally shown loyalty and respect. The butler, Williams, had been with her for many years and despite giving each other notice from time to time they understood each other well.

Once I had the temerity to ask Williams – always a good friend to us – to put two shillings on a Derby horse for me. It won and in my jubilation I failed to keep my mouth shut. Williams was given a severe scolding for leading the young astray and was given notice. The bet had been put through the good offices of a van delivery boy, and this off-the-course betting was strictly illegal then. After a bit Granny had had her say and human curiosity took over. 'Now tell me, Williams, how exactly does one place a bet?' The notice, of course, was forgotten.

Granny had a devoted personal maid and companion called Miss Eden, who was a wizened middle aged person who seldom smiled. She looked after Granny's wardrobe and prepared and mended her clothes. Her care for Granny was such that when a young godchild of my father's fell off her pony and broke her arm all the sympathy she got from Miss Eden was 'be quite, child, Granny is having her afternoon sleep' instead of the help and concern she needed.

Sundays were very much special days and morning prayers in the church across the park was a solemn event. Wearing our best clothes, a blue serge suit in my case, we would walk through the park past old mature oak trees and cows chewing the cud to the village church with its bells ringing a change to a rhythm which sounded like 'come to church' which is how we used to interpret it. On the way we would meet local lads who would touch their quiffs to Aunt Bea who might quiz them and sometimes tell them that they should doff their caps properly on saying 'good morning' to her. Meanwhile Granny had been driven by her chauffeur, Mr. Longland, to the service. If the weather was bad we, too, would be taken by car.

Inside the church the choir would sit at the west end led by Aunt Bea, and the organ which was adjacent to the choir was played by my Aunt Cis and the power was provided by a hand bellows worked by an under gardener. On one occasion it emitted dreadful groans and squeaks when a mouse was caught in the works. The villagers and servants would sit in the nave; dark clothes, hats and black gloves were the order of the day for the servants. In the chancel were the seats for the family, their guests, and their friends facing across the aisle. To us small children the morning service would seem to be interminably long and the pews hard and uncomfortable. Restlessness or talking or whispering was severely frowned upon. The sermons would take at least twenty minutes and at the end would come the final hymn and the collection. Afterwards the walk back across the park with the prospect of a good lunch to come was a blessed relief. When my father was there he would read the lessons clearly and intelligently having studied the texts beforehand with his scholarly mind.

The great festivals of the year were memorable occasions and this was especially so at Christmas. The house would be full of members of the family and guests, and there would be great feelings of expectation with promises of presents and feasting.

In the so-called music room a large Christmas tree would stand in the centre decorated with lights and tinsel with small parcels suspended from it and larger ones stacked at its base.

On Christmas Eve the children from the village school would be grouped at the juncture of the inner and outer halls to sing carols before receiving presents and a meal with the sort of goodies which appeal to children. But first, the apprehensive teacher would get her eager flock into order, and then after giving a middle C on a tuning fork would launch her charges into the traditional carols. We, of the house, would applaud and then help to serve the food.

Nowadays this kind of thing might be described as elitism, social injustice, class inequality or discrimination and conde-scension, but as children we accepted life as it came and took it to be the order of things. In church we might have sung the hymn which includes the words 'the rich man in his castle and the poor man at his gate. God made them high and lowly, and ordered their estate'.

However, these thoughts did not bother us as children and I had friends of my own age about the farm and grounds and could feel more at ease with them than with some of my relations.

As bedtime approached our excitement would rise with the hanging up of an old black stocking of my mother's for the eagerly anticipated arrival of Father Christmas. We were not supposed to see him come into the room, and still awake, we would snuggle under the bedclothes when the door to the bedroom was opened quietly, and we would know that he had arrived. Then we would sleep until morning when we would be wakened by Williams or one of the servants who would carefully fold our untidily discarded clothes and make up the fire in the room. Then would come the joys of emptying the stocking with the help of parents and sisters. Always there was an orange at the bottom.

Then, after breakfast, we would get ready for church with our thoughts on the Christmas lunch to come and later in the day the Christmas tree with the handing out of presents. The service would be a cheerful one with the lessons from familiar bits of the Bible read by my father. On a fine day the walk back from church to the house would be a needed breath of fresh air in the day's busy programme, though occasionally an aunt might quiz one on the contents of the sermon we had just heard usually with little attention.

Christmas lunch was the formal family event of the day with aunts, uncles and cousins assembled in the morning room waiting for the large double mahogany doors leading into the dining room to open. There was an order of precedence as we went in with Granny leading the way. When all were assembled she would ask one of us to say grace 'For what we are about to receive may the Lord make us truly thankful: amen'. Then with a shuffling of chairs we would sit down to a five course Christmas lunch.

The table was resplendent with the family silver, galleons in full sail, candlesticks, silver horses and dogs and other ornaments.

An enormous turkey would be ceremonially carved by Williams who loved these occasions, and we would watch out for our helping with all the appurtenances to be served to us. But the real treat was to come in the rich Christmas pudding which we knew contained traditional charms and coins. The charms included a thimble, a button, a slipper, a ring, and the coins were threepenny pieces and sixpences. Williams would see that we children got a coin, though this could mean having a second helping. Usually we had helped to stir the Christmas pudding and see that the charms were included when we were staying at Sacombe earlier in the autumn. After the meal, someone would be asked to say grace – 'for what we have received may the Lord make us truly thankful: amen'. Once a somewhat rumbustious rugger-playing cousin of ours from Scotland said 'for what we have received may the good Lord deliver us'. Alec who was a rebel and disliked formality was asked to leave.

The summons would then come for the youngest bachelor to open the heavy doors of the dining room leading to the morning room for Granny to leave in state. Then there would be a lull in the festivities until tea with a rich Christmas cake followed by the handing out of presents around the Christmas tree.

Inevitably all the excitement and rich food would take its toll in the aftermath, and malaise, including asthma in my case, would ensue, and Nanny would be kept busy nursing us back onto our feet. When I was a bit older I would hope to be well enough to go with my father on the Boxing Day shoot.

On one occasion I was asked by my Aunt Bea to go for a walk with a pernickety lady who I and the other children disliked, and so miss the shoot. I soon got into trouble for taking her through muddy fields and facing her with stiles she could not negotiate easily. This led to a severe ticking-off from my Aunt Bea and I was given to understand that I was rude, vulgar and nasty with no respect for my elders and betters, and that my prospects in this world were wretched to say the least.

Apologetic and crestfallen, I slunk away to plan my revenge for this terrible scolding. At a quiet moment I crept into my aunt's bedroom and emptied a generous measure of Eno's Fruit Salts into her chamberpot hoping it would fizz when nature was relieved in the middle of the night. The trick, meant only as a practical joke, worked only too well. Next morning there was a hush in the house and we were told that Aunt Bea was ill and that the doctor had been summoned to call, and this he did being let in through a side door or tradesman's entrance.

Solemn voices soon made it apparent that the diagnosis was proving to be a difficult one. This made me feel very guilty and uncomfortable, so that I was driven to confess what I had done. Inevitably and rightly, I was given a good scolding and made to feel that I was bound for the nether regions unless I could reform my ways.

I was seldom happy or at ease in Sacombe House, but I have happy memories of the farm, the woods, and the countryside with the park where specimen oaks grew with rabbit holes around their roots. Mr Hale the gamekeeper was my special friend, and as soon as possible after arrival I would make for his cottage situated in a spinney approached only by a rough track. I would go into the warm parlour with its wood fired stove and be given cocoa or chocolate to drink and a cake.

Mr Hale and his family of wife and two sons would then regale me with all the latest news about how the game was doing, how the organized shoots had fared, or the problem of poachers. He was a genius with gun dogs and renowned for his training methods. The dogs would give one a rapturous welcome with the uncritical joy and affection dogs can show. He could leave a dog guarding his game bag or perhaps fodder for reared pheasants while he went off to inspect some coverts, and it would never move until he returned.

Hale was not very literate but he had a gift of expressing himself directly and with humour, his stories being punctuated by such expressions as 'cor love a duck' accompanied by hearty laughter. He was a survivor of the First World War and had been a sniper until taken prisoner in an enemy offensive, but he had managed to escape back to his own lines. He taught me to shoot, first with a 410 shot-gun and, later, with a 12 bore. He was strict on safety drill and on more than one occasion I heard him use army language on a cousin of mine who was the eldest son of my uncle who owned the shooting rights, when my cousin Alec had transgressed the safety drill.

I spent long hours with him on his rounds and he would teach me to spot pheasants or partridges sitting on their nests in the hedgerows when I would never have seen them on my own. I disliked the gamekeepers' larders which were where the corpses of vermin were tied up to hedges; there were rats, owls, stoats, weasels, crows and magpies among others; but trapping and shooting so-called vermin was part of his job.

Foxes were a different matter, as they were the prey of the local hunt and enjoyed a special place in the lives of the 'county set'. Nevertheless, they could wreak havoc among the game especially the pheasants most of which had been hand reared. Hale let me in the secret that the time to shoot foxes was in the early morning when most people were asleep in bed. He promised that I could go with him if I could leave the house undetected.

I had often strolled in the garden and woods before breakfast, so it was not difficult to make an early start and to meet him in Home Wood. It turned out to be an exciting sport needing field-craft to outwit the wily fox creeping noiselessly through the woodland tracks. The death of so beautiful a creature was to be regretted, and the body had to be buried before any of the household dogs could find it. I returned to the house for breakfast with a good appetite and a delicious sense of adventure and guilt.

My grandmother died when I was about fourteen and the house and farm were sold, the shooting rights passing into the hands of a syndicate; but when staying with other relations in the neighbourhood I could walk over to Hale's cottage to hear his news. Always loyal to the gentry who employed him, provided they kept to the traditional country codes, he was unhappy with the syndicate, which was composed of *nouveau riche* business men who knew little about how to handle sporting guns safely. One of them was found to be using ball cartridge and all the time bets were being laid on the amount of game likely to be bagged.

When the war started Hale became a key man in the local Home Guard and had the Germans invaded they would have suffered heavily on his patch.

To call him one of nature's gentlemen would not be an idle cliché in his case. He was loyal and highly professional at his work which he enjoyed so much. He had a great sense of humour and taught my cousins and myself how to enjoy country sport and how to handle sporting guns with safety. He also had respect for the quarry, and after a big shoot I would go round with him to collect any wounded birds or hares.

Later in life, when I had learned more about living animals and birds, my taste for killing left me and I sold the Purdey gun which I inherited from my father, but not before I had enjoyed days of rough shooting and wild-fowling when the bag was usually a small one and destined for the family pot.

The big formal shoots with beaters driving the game towards the guns awaiting them were exciting to me when I accompanied my father on them. The sight of the corpses of birds and hares set out on display at the end of the day to gratify the hunting instincts of my uncle's wealthy guests did not appeal to me. What I really enjoyed was being in the woods and country-side and seeing something of the farming and other activities through the changing seasons. In those days harvesting, hay-making and ploughing were not as mechanised as they are today, though one enterprising farmer in the area used steam traction engines instead of Shire horses on his larger fields.

There was a home farm run by my Aunt Cis, a large lady, always happiest in tweeds and pork pie hats directing the farm, or in winter hunting on large horses side-saddle. She was also a competent musician and played the violin well if not with distinction. She loved to sponsor young female players, some of whom owed her a great deal. She was not interested in men though she was fond of my father in a possessive way which made her jealous of my mother for deserting her musical female entourage and marrying my father.

Aunt Cis was my godmother and though I seldom felt at ease with her, there remains much that I have to thank her for including the farm with its herd of dewy-eyed Jersey cows which had been mated with the resident bull, usually a fero-cious and active creature exercised daily by a farm hand wielding a long pole attached to the bull by a ring fixed in its nose. Near the farm was the dairy where the very rich cream was separated out, and the butter was churned.

Fishing was a sport enjoyed by both my Aunt Bea and my Aunt Cis, who before the last war would spend a month or two in a farmhouse in Scotland near Taynuilt. She drove an open four-seater Austin car over rough and remote roads to sea lochs and places of interest. My father and myself would be invited to join her, though my mother was never asked to stay there. Those days in the Highlands captured my imagination and since then my family and I have had many happy holidays there.

Chapter 3

Public School and University

My father was delighted that I had been accepted to go to his old school, Sherborne, if not to his old house. He was always loyal to his past and to the education which had led him to become a qualified doctor. So off I went with other new boys dressed in a ridiculous and uncomfortable school uniform surmounted by a flattish straw boater with a ribbon round it in the appropriate house colours.

There have been many accounts of what life was like in a pre-war public school, and as with many of the authors I found it a hateful and traumatic experience in the main, though there were some mitigating times. Survival was particularly difficult if one had any physical disability especially something like asthma which, in the eyes of some, carried with it the aura of moral weakness or lack of moral fibre: a missing limb or some obvious disfigurement was more acceptable.

The only person I can think of whom I have really hated at the personal level was my housemaster. He was a large man with a nervous tic which twisted his mouth into hideous grimaces. His great ambition was for his house to excel at games, drill and physical fitness. He had a terrifying temper backed up by a ready use of the cane. I kept as low a profile as I could and lived from day to day counting the time to the end of term and to the holidays.

Bullying among the boys was rife, but being tall for my age this did not bother me very much. We lived in spartan discomfort, the day starting after the dreaded ringing of a hand bell followed with a cold shower and press-ups to ensure that we were awake and geared-up for action.

This kind of conditioning had its good points in that discomforts when they were encountered from time to time later on in life were easily met without much stress, and I am thinking of occasions while working in wartime hospitals and in the R.A.F. The worst feature for me was the almost total lack of privacy at school. The outside world appeared to be so free compared to our existence, and I envied the delivery boys and working lads for what I thought I saw as their self reliance and the supposed safety of their homes and families, where they could make many decisions for themselves.

Again, like in Sparta of old, we were taught to look upon girls as being inferior. The precincts of the girls' school were strictly out of bounds as if a sort of *cordon sanitaire* had been drawn round it. Once I saw a crocodile of girls being given an abrupt command to do an about turn and hurry off in the other direction because boys of our school had been spotted in the street.

Needless to say this sort of thing gave the stimulus for the more adventurous boys to indulge in some risky exploits in stalking the girls, though these were innocent enough games. The whole system must have encouraged any homosexual tendencies among the boys, and this was probably exacerbated by the fag system which gave rise, on occasions, to favourites and heroes, though generally it was hated by the junior boys who looked forward to becoming senior themselves and able to order others about.

Once, when sitting next to the housemaster's wife at lunch, eating as second course a disgusting junket dusted with grated nutmeg, she held forth on the moral excellence and cleanness of the school. I agreed with her politely without knowing the purport of this homily.

Dislike of the system made me think of ways whereby I might assert myself without running the risk of condign retribution. The opportunity came when I was told that the time for confirmation was approaching, and that those of the right age would be confirmed by the bishop in the abbey.

I had been lectured in a desultory way on the catechism and the creed. I had never understood either of them, though that had not bothered me much. I had been told that I was to think of God first, the school next, and self last. But when it came to affirming in public and before an audience that I believed in dogmas which did not make sense to me, I jibbed and refused to be involved. This disconcerted my housemaster and he gave me a private lecture on the subject of letting down the side, and the prospect of being consigned to outer darkness. Worst of all, my refusal would upset the house statistics of religious success. I knew that this heinous crime could not be dealt with by the usual sort of punishments for supposed misdemeanours.

Regrettably, this upset my parents, particularly my mother, but since then I have considered it wrong to declare solemnly that one believes something if one does not do so, as that would mean telling oneself a lie which might catch one out later. Over the years I had been taught much of the Old Testament and the New Testament and in the happy atmosphere of Château D'Oex I had accepted Christian teaching easily if uncritically.

A spirit of rivalry and competition between the houses was fostered to the extent that my housemaster discouraged the formation of friendships with the juniors of other houses whom we met in class; this was, of course, ineffective.

The headmaster of the whole school was a weak man who, I realize in retrospect, was suffering from the effects of his war service. He was really a kindly and humane man who, among other things, abolished boxing as part of physical education; but he was not popular with the masters or boys, and at one school occasion he received the slow handclap when he appeared, instead of the enthusiastic applause leaders are supposed to get.

At that time the British Empire was taken for granted, and the school prided itself on educating future soldiers, administrators, and others destined for overseas service of various kinds.

Many old boys gave unselfish service despite the narrowness of the attitudes the school sought to inculcate through a sort of brain washing. As an instance of the latter, at a summer half-term celebration some of us junior boys were dragooned into playing the role of Indian rioters at a time when civil disobedience was spreading in that country. The rioters were, naturally, dispersed by seniors dressed as sahibs and Indian police, who bravely upheld authority.

However, it was all enjoyable as an opportunity to act the rebel legitimately in play, but the whole show epitomised the narrow bad taste of a school which made no attempt to show us any other side of a problem so vitally important to many people whose lives were lacking in hope or privilege.

The attitude towards the underdogs in this country also smacked of condescension. It was taken for granted that we were to be trained as future leaders, and it went without saying who were to be the led whether they liked the prospect or not. Every summer boys from an East End London club were invited for a weekend of games and entertainment, but generally speaking the barriers were never down, though some old boys went on later in life to do good charitable work in poor areas.

As always, there were some pleasant compensations made all the more enjoyable by contrast with the usual course of life. The country around was superb, and we were allowed to bicycle within a small radius of the school. Once in the quiet lanes away from the main roads, it was possible to explore further afield and to enjoy the quiet, dreamy Dorset villages so remote from the hassle of school.

Some boys were more daring and adventurous, as I found out much later on when I met an old boy who was the Intelligence Officer of an R.A.F. station where I was a Medical Officer. A bit of a lady's man he had had his early instruction in the pleasures of sex from a widow living in some remote old-world cottage who found some consolation in instructing the young in these activities.

Another pleasure was found in O.T.C. field days when we would go into the country and play innocent war games, stalking the enemy along hedges or charging the enemy's position. With the country lore I had learned from my game-keeper friend Mr Hale I was able to pass the time away enjoying the bird and insect life around me while awaiting action. The annual O.T.C. inspection by a visiting general was a bit of an ordeal as it meant standing at attention for a long time before being appraised by the great man in a brief but glassy eyeball-to-eyeball encounter. There was also marching and drill while the execrable bugle and drum band played martial tunes. At the end the great man would deliver a patriotic homily.

The best breaks of all came in the expeditions organized by the archaeological society. The masters who ran it were keen and knowledgeable historians, and they took us by coach to prehistoric sites, and to famous places like Old Sarum, Bath, Glastonbury and many others. We also visited the Wookey Hole caves being allowed to go into parts not then open to the public. These outings have left me with some very pleasant memories.

Having grown out of the more junior group into the middle ranks of the house, I could look forward to some amelioration of living conditions with the prospect of a shared study, a freedom from fagging, and to have other minor privileges.

Then it was that I contracted bronchopneumonia and was sent to the school sick bay. There were no antibiotics in those days and my asthma became much worse. The school doctor was an elderly, sporting medico keen on hunting and dogs. He had bandy legs reputed by the boys to be the result of a riding accident when bones had been broken and then badly set. One day he came to see me when I was very ill. He was accompanied by his spaniel who jumped on my bed and began to lick my face when I was too weak to push it off me. My father was contacted and he fetched me home in a hired car much to my relief. I recovered slowly, and my parents wisely decided that I should not return to Sherborne school.

I was taken to see a variety of doctors and specialists, and had a variety of treatments then in vogue, some of which were distinctly unpleasant. One Harley Street consultant said he thought I ought to aim at chicken farming as a career, though chicken feathers and the dust and dirt associated with hens we now know to be the worst possible atmosphere for an asthmatic with allergy to be in; and, of course, my parents and myself dismissed such advice.

What helped me most at that stage was going to a gymnasium run by a Mr Percy Sage an ex-army N.C.O. and his assistant a Mr Smith another ex-N.C.O. with war experience. Besides running classes for schools, with the help of a blind pianist, they undertook remedial work and individual training work-outs for athletes of various kinds. The atmosphere was one of vigour and fun, and my health and confidence soon returned thanks to their skills and their cheerful optimism.

For a term or two I went to a tutor's establishment to continue with my education. The instruction was good particularly as we got individual attention, but some of the other students were somewhat odd in ways that I could not understand at the time. So with the prospect of winter and the annual London smogs, my parents arranged for me to return to Mr and Mrs Kitchin at the Châlet du Vallon at Château D'Oex to be coached up for the school certificate examination, the stepping stone to university and higher education.

To return to the place I loved was the best tonic my long suffering parents could have given me, and once again as I sat in the electric and clean M.O.B. train going from Montreux into the mountains with the smell of the evergreen woods and the sounds of the cowbells in the meadows I felt I could face the future with confidence and hope.

Once again I would be able to sit in the sun on the garden steps with Verney in shorts, but this time helping me with the letters of Cicero. His knowledge and enthusiasm brought them to life and made me enjoy Latin literature in general.

A young, cheery graduate from Oxford called Mr Peacock taught us mathematics and chemistry. One of his experiments went awry and chlorine was released which put me into bed, coughing, for a day or two. He also fancied himself as a climber and introduced some of us to elementary rope work and mountain lore. After one trip with him he treated us to beer; I had never tasted this before and thought it revolting, but being thirsty after our sally into the mountains I continued to drink it, finding that the taste improved with every sip.

When winter came I was able to do some expeditions on skis, and on one of these we had to take shelter for several hours from a storm. We had a Swiss guide with us and he made some rich soup to which he added some dried fungi, and when the storm abated and the visibility improved he led us safely back to the valley over rough snow from a minor avalanche. This, too, was a useful lesson on respect for the forces of nature.

At last in July the time came for some of us to take the school certificate. We were joined by other candidates from other English tutorial establishments. The weather was hot and sultry with thunder rolling intermittently round the mountains. Thanks to the Kitchins I passed this hurdle without too much difficulty.

It was at about this time that the Kitchins lost their eldest son in a motor cycle accident in England where he was a student at Cambridge. This caused much sorrow to all who knew the family and some of us had got to know him well with his friendliness to us and his adventurous nature. Château D'Oex and the Kitchins left me with a host of happy memories which have not faded as have the more difficult experiences I had at boarding schools, which over some years gave rise to night-mares that I was returning to Sherborne again as a junior when my friends were now senior.

But one awakes from nightmares to recognise them for what they are and to turn ones attention to the happier times such as I enjoyed with the Kitchins. I kept in touch with them until the last war during which I thought about them and the beauty of the Alps very often when it was a great help to recall visually and verbally so much which I had come to value as an antidote to difficult experiences.

It was decided that I should go in for a medical career which in those days meant passing three M.B. examinations over the next four or five years. The first M.B. was the equivalent of the modern A levels, and to study for this I was to go to St. Bartholomew's Hospital in London to do physics, chemistry biology.

My parents had moved house to Addison Road in Kensington. It was a nice and spacious detached house with a walled garden which gave my mother and the family much pleasure as the house in Hill Street had not even got a yard of open space except for the narrow drawing room balcony. I had also reached the age when I could have a driving licence and I had some driving lessons and some elementary instruction in car maintenance.

My father never drove, but used London taxis. When my eldest sister was old enough to have a licence we acquired our first family car, but for the moment I had the use of London public transport to take me to and from work and on expeditions of exploration of the city and its environs.

The teaching was good, and in particular I remember the lectures of Professor Hopwood who was a physicist. In a calm and impressive way he would put any difficult pupil in his place. He was a pioneer in X-ray treatments and bore the scars on his hands which had resulted from some of his experiments. When I left, his parting advice was 'remember moderation in all things even in being moderate' an aphorism I have passed on to patients and others since then, and only recently somebody reminded me that I had said this to them twenty-five years ago.

The professor of chemistry had a penchant for the dramatic and he loved to emphasize some of his themes with smoke, flames and minor explosions at the end of his lectures. Biology lectures were apt to be chaotic as students ragged the professor as he read out his sermons from written texts of his own composition. Most of the students were working for the London M.B. and their syllabus was different in minor details to the Cambridge one. For some reason we were required to dissect cockroaches and this meant going down into the boiler rooms with torches to capture them.

I have a few clear memories of that period. One student was an interesting Norwegian much older than the rest of us. He had been a sisal farmer in Kenya, and at one stage had been invited to Ethiopia by King Haile Selassie to introduce his farming methods to that country. He had been to exotic banquets in the palace and had had some unusual and wonderful experiences which made our daily rounds seem humdrum. The hurdle of the first M.B. was taken successfully, and about then I went to Cambridge to take the Caius College entrance examination which included a Latin paper.

In the autumn of 1933 I went up to Caius College, Cambridge where my father had been a student also studying medicine. For the first year I had rooms at the top of one of the old buildings forming one side of a quadrangle. They were cold and draughty in the bitter winter weather with the winds driving off the fenlands, and it was necessary to go down several flights of stairs and across the quadrangle to get a bath. Heating still depended on coal fires, though if I remember correctly, there was a gas ring on which we did simple cookery.

Dinner in Hall was an obligation and dressed in academic undergraduate gowns we sat at long tables overlooked by the top table occupied by the dons and sometimes the Master. Scholars said Latin graces before and after the meals. These were pleasant traditional occasions linking us with the college past and its history of teaching and research.

After the first year I went into lodgings in Jesus Lane. They overlooked a green patch of common adjoining the river Cam, and being away from the centre of Cambridge they were quiet. The landlady was a pleasant motherly person and I lived in comfort.

Going up to Cambridge brought home to me that I was now an adult and my future would depend on my own efforts and judgement. There were all sorts of pressures on students to join societies or groups dedicated to doubtful ends. By nature and experience I was diffident and shy of committing myself to any of them. In particular, religious organizations were keen to gather in new recruits.

I had never been confirmed and was suspicious of attempts to get myself too involved in what I did not understand. A keen young clergyman, a member of the then fashionable Oxford Group, had been asked by my mother to give me private religious instruction when I had left Sherborne School. He had been earnest with intense dark eyes which sought to nail me with his gaze, as with facial contortions he had told me, his fingers clasping and unclasping, that moral strength and cleanliness were to be obtained by spiritual exercise and prayer, like physical fitness was to be obtained by training, courage and manliness.

As physical exercise was apt to give me asthma this analogy was not well received by me, and fortunately the sessions stopped due to lack of progress or perhaps obstinacy on my part. The Dean of Caius at the time was a learned man, but he chose to regale us at the missionary breakfast for freshmen with his war experiences besides his brand of theology.

We had to wear attenuated white surplices in the college chapel which made me feel self conscious and absurd. Anyway, I was going through a materialistic phase of life with so much of my attention on anatomy and physiology. I doubt whether I was an atheist then or later as my mind often returned to my experiences at Château D'Oex, and I was ever conscious of the love and support I had received from my parents, the Kitchins and in particular my godmother Aunt Kit. They had shown me the positive side of life and had given me the hope and confidence I needed. It is curious that their deaths left me with not so much a feeling of loss as one of deepened gratitude for all they have given me. If heaven means a continued existence in some form and they are part of it that would be promise enough for me.

The anatomy course began with a lecture followed by an introduction to the dissecting room where twenty or so bodies were laid out on slabs ready for us to dissect with scalpels and forceps. I, like most of the others, had never seen a dead body before as our generation, unlike most of the previous ones, had had so much of the facts of birth, life and death hidden from us.

The first time I had seen a woman's naked body was when I saw one as a corpse on a slab. This was disturbing emotionally to start with, but there was work to be done and the interest of anatomy and its intricacies soon kept our minds occupied.

The professor of anatomy was Professor Harris, a robust character, who did not tolerate fools easily, and he was a splendid teacher. Once, in an end of term practical examination, he asked me about some artery and its relations to other structures. My answer did not please him, and in a mood of desperation I replied that in the specimen I had been working on it was as I had said. He went over to my specimen, and found that I had described some rare anomaly, and he spent the rest of the viva giving me a fascinating talk on how it might have come about, ending by saying 'it's much better to see for yourself than to believe what you are told'; a good piece of advice which has stood me in good stead.

Once, in a lecture, some students tried to create a diversion with a stupid prank letting down a large model spider from the ceiling onto the lecturer's desk. Glaring at the guilty parties who were fairly easily identified he gave an extempore dissertation on the subject of Kidloids, Childikens and Edicles. The Kidloids had the mental and emotional development appropriate to five year olds, the Childikens covered the next ten years or so, and the Edicles were those at the university who, lacking much experience, had the solutions for all the problems and expected to be admired and adulated. These are useful categories to describe those with adult bodies but with retarded emotional development.

The physiology department was in the hands of Professor Sir Joseph Barcroft a great man and a great character whose lectures were always well attended and full of memorable anecdotes. On one occasion the door behind the lecturer's table was flung open in the middle of the professor's lecture and a wild looking figure appeared unshaven and with tousled hair and shouted in a loud voice 'I have seen the face of God'.

Turning round to face the intruder the professor said 'that sounds to be most interesting. Now as so many of us are here together perhaps you would tell us what it looked like.' The reply came 'like the molecule of H_2O_2'. This turned out to be a good example of gross caffeine intoxication. The research worker had been spending long hours on some experiment which had gone on through the night. He had kept himself awake by sipping coffee brewed over a bunsen burner.

There was a lot of work to get through, and much of our time was taken up in the laboratories. Medical students had to go up for a long vacation term to keep up with the syllabus. These long vacation terms were very pleasant times. There was an air of informality and one was not rushed. Many tourists and visitors from abroad were about, and some societies then, as now, would hire accommodation for their summer conventions. One year there was a gathering of members of the Oxford Group in Caius. They were a fervent but jolly lot eager to confess their sins real or imagined.

It was also possible to attend some clinical ward rounds at Addenbrooke's Hospital, and though at first feeling squeamish at some of the procedures I soon lost any doubts I may have had about being able to do medicine.

Because I was still subject to asthma attacks and wheezing on exertion I missed out on many of the college activities I would have like to have enjoyed. I could manage tennis and sometimes squash if I took ephedrine tablets in advance. I even tried hockey and could just about manage that until I was promoted on trial to the college first eleven, but then the game was taken too seriously for me and afraid of letting down the side I gave up the sport.

Then I joined the Trinity Foot Beagles. These outings I thoroughly enjoyed with my love of and interest in the English countryside. I could go easy when necessary or take a rest until the ephedrine had worked when I started to wheeze, but often I would get a second wind and be able to keep up well. We used to meet at farms or country houses and see something of rural life and work. In those days factory farming had not been developed and hedges around fields were still intact.

In the summer I took long bicycle rides exploring the villages in the neighbourhood and on one occasion going as far away as Wisbech. Cycling to Newmarket to see the horses on the gallops was another pleasure.

Then there was the river Cam. With a friend who was to become a distinguished surgeon we would paddle upstream to Granchester and beyond in Rob Roy canoes and penetrate up small tributaries with reeds where we could observe the wild life at close quarters if we kept quiet: there were moorhens with their families, water rats and grass-snakes, and insects including dragonflies and butterflies among others. On the way we would swim in Granchester Pool.

The more socially inclined concentrated on the punts in which they would take their girl friends along the Backs. In spite of having sisters I was shy of girls and always conscious that any bout of wheezing would be unromantic and absurd.

I used to enjoy some of the debates in the Union though I never took much part in them. At that time it was smart to be left wing or a supporter of the Communist Party. Tragically, the Spanish Civil War was to entice some young idealists to volunteer to fight and some like John Cornford to lose their lives. My outlook was right wing in theory, but I think that what put me off left wing politics is that I saw them as a threat to the ideals of my parents and to my own future security. However, humour and levity mitigated some of the abrasive side of politics.

On one occasion some of the 'reds' managed to remove the fuses in a cinema showing a film about the navy. The opposition got wind of this, and led by an ex-service pipe band marched on the cinema which was situated by the river Cam and routed the Marxists throwing some of them into the water.

Another rag was perpetrated by a cousin of mine who, as a brilliant linguist and actor, addressed a League of Nations meeting in the guise of a Russian delegate. He had packed the back of the hall with friends let into the plot including non university people. Platitudes in a guttural foreign accent flowed from the stout, unshaven figure as he thumped the Union Jack covered table. Uproar ensued as cheers, wolf whistles, and the singing of the Red Flag erupted from the back of the hall.

One day I joined the Judo club. A friend of mine had persuaded me to go along with him and watch the training. Men were throwing each other around on the mat in a hair raising way with resounding thumps. I was impressed but thought it was not the sort of violent activity for me.

However, in a lull, the professor of this art suggested that I might like to try. He was a large amiable man with a benign smile on his face: I have forgotten his name but it was something like J.J. Knonshiel. Despite his hefty thick set frame he was remarkably agile and quick in his reactions. I tried to decline his invitation, but was told that all I had to do was to lie on the mat and a small man who was a rowing eight cox would stop me getting up. So I did what had been suggested and found that I could hardly move from the hold down, let alone get up. My self esteem had been dented and I joined.

It turned out to be a cheerful club and I learned some useful tricks in the way of hold downs which had their uses later on when dealing with drunken casualties. J.J. had a fund of good stories to tell us. A friend of mine also joined and once or twice we put on a show to impress any visitors. Bob who stayed on at Cambridge for a fourth year went on to be in the University Judo team.

Another recreation was horse riding. The mother of a student friend of mine kept some horses at Histon and I used to cycle over there and enjoy some hacking through the countryside. At the time of the summer examinations I would go for a ride before breakfast forgetting my worries about anatomy and physiology. I would arrive at the examination rooms feeling healthy and robust when some of my colleagues were anxious and drawn from last minute swatting the previous night. I am sure that horse riding contributed to my being able to get a good second class degree.

I had enjoyed Cambridge and was sad at the prospect of leaving to enter the last stage of medical training at St. Bartholomew's Hospital when I would be living at home in

London. Another pleasant period of my life had ended, I had become an adult and had started to think about what sort of niche I would find in life to earn a living.

Times were restless with the Spanish Civil War, the rise of Hitler and Mussolini and the threats of communism as the answer to poverty and deprivation which were obvious in such events as the hunger marches. Of course, I was too naive to realise that groups like the Cambridge Apostles were already scheming to attain influence and power in society and the state. There were few serious politicians among the more earthy medical students. Having a good measure of privacy I was able to control my asthma and by guile and dissimulation avoid it from coming too much to the notice of others. I felt this to be an aid to self confidence and independence.

Chapter 4

Clinical Student

Having done well enough in the Cambridge Medical Tripos examination to be exempted from taking the second M.B. I became a clinical student at my father's old hospital St. Bartholomew's in the City of London close to Smithfield meat market. Apart from attending some clinical rounds at Addenbrooke's Hospital in Cambridge during my last long vacation term, I was now introduced to meeting real patients for the first time.

The history of Barts and its service to the city of London goes back to the twelfth century. Like so many institutions dedicated to helping people it was inspired at its beginnings by a far sighted individual, in this case a monk, Rahere. Barts has produced a long line of distinguished surgeons and physicians and still does so. When I was there the senior staff were not only leading men in their own fields, but they were great characters as well so that their teaching was for ever to be remembered linked to a vivid recall of their persons.

The Dean was Sir Girling Ball a large, ebullient surgeon. His lecture on gallstones was illustrated by a jar in which was preserved a large gall-bladder with stones which had been extracted from himself. Holding the jar affectionately against the appropriate part of his belly he recounted vividly from first hand what the patient had felt and experienced. He called his Rolls Royce the scrotum as it contained the two Balls – there were no women students there in those days.

46

There was Sir Geoffrey Keynes a pioneer of much in surgery and the use of blood transfusion. He was one of the earliest users of radium needles in the treatment of some types of cancer. He was a great showman and loved demonstrating his methods to visiting surgeons. His literary interests made him into the leading authority on William Blake, and this combined with a knowledge of the arts and the theatre, led him to help produce the masque Job. Many years later I met his then registrar now a leading surgeon. He told me that he had been offered the part of Jehovah which only meant walking across the stage in a dignified way accompanied by music and sit on the heavenly throne. Unfortunately, my friend refused the part, but as I said to him there are not many of us asked to act as Jehovah.

I was also a dresser on the firm of the surgeon John Hosford. A surgeon to his finger tips, his no nonsense approach to solving problems and his clarity of mind made the subject enthralling. Often I would stay on late into the evening to watch him and his registrars deal with the intake of emergency cases, when I would be allowed to assist in a minor capacity. I can remember his fuming one evening as a Christian Scientist refused to give her permission for an emergency operation. She eventually went into coma; he operated, and she recovered.

However, before becoming a dresser on a surgical or medical firm we were started off in the casualty department where we were presented with a large variety of clinical material ranging from the serious and difficult to the trivial. Among the latter, as I thought, was a tough meat porter from Smithfield market wanting his ears to be syringed. I was deputed to do this job and conscientiously got the water at the right temperature and the syringe at the right angle before starting very gently on my first minor medical procedure as laid down in the clinical hand book.

I began the operation carefully and nothing happened. Then the wax plug began to move and the patient with an exclamation of 'watch it mate' collapsed unconscious onto the floor bumping his head heavily on the metal table on the way down.

I felt that I had done something terrible as I knelt down beside him checking for signs of life. He was a large, florid man and so the question as to how to get him off the floor from under the table and onto a couch posed problems. To my immense relief he came round, sat up rubbing his head where he had bumped it, and apologised saying 'sorry, doc, I meant to tell yer it always does this to me; if I lie down for this I'm alright'.

The meat market provided us with some gory gashes caused by carelessly wielded or ill directed cleavers and knives used to dismember the carcases, and we soon became proficient at stitching the wounds. Fractures and more serious cases were admitted or treated by qualified house doctors whom we regarded with envy and awe wondering if we ourselves could ever pass our examinations and achieve their positions.

There were courses of lectures and demonstrations to be attended and many hours were spent in the library and doing written and reading work at home. Sometimes I would go to the Wellcome Pathology and Medical History Museum then in the Euston Road and enjoy the imaginative display of specimens.

The next stage in working with patients was doing a clerkship in the septic wards. Before the days of antibiotics people unlucky enough to contract osteomyelitis which is a chronic infection of bones would lie for many weeks with their wounds exposed hoping that natural processes would eventually lead to healing. Many were dreadful cases to see and sometimes the ward sister would use an antiseptic scent spray to mitigate the smell as the deep and open wounds were displayed to us.

Just before I began my clinical studies at St Barts, a Mr Nelson who was a young and brilliant surgeon contracted septicemia in the course of operating on a patient with a septic condition. He got pricked in the hand with a piece of infected bone or a needle. This resulted in a severe local infection which was treated by amputation to prevent its spread. Despite this operation, which would have meant the end of his career as a surgeon, he died. In those days to say of anyone that they had a nasty infection could result in the sort of anxieties people now experience when they hear the word cancer mentioned.

Tuberculosis was another common infection with acute and deadly outcomes in many cases such as when it infected the coverings of the brain and spinal cord, or when it spread rapidly in the lungs. We would examine patients including looking down their throats causing them to gag or cough if we were not careful, and then later peer through a microscope at specimens of their spit to find it swarming with tubercle bacteria. In one's imagination one could wonder whether any of the bugs had lodged in one's own lungs.

The venereal disease department was also an education in more senses than one. Most of us had come from relatively sheltered middle class backgrounds where sexual problems and peccadilloes were not mentioned in the way they are now. Some of us were shocked at seeing cases of late syphilis with disastrous complications like tabes dorsalis and general paralysis of the insane. Patients would queue up in the clinic for us to administer a preparation of arsenic or bismuth by injection. As far as I can remember there was very little counselling of the unfortunate patients, but hospitals were then voluntary establishments and money was much shorter than it is now.

As far as I can remember, we had little or no practical experience of treating women patients with V.D. though when doing gynaecology we saw some of the effects of pelvic sepsis and the results of back street abortions. A dedicated genito-urinary surgeon, Kenneth Walker, was our teacher in V.D. and genito-urinary medicine. Among his skills was ability to do quick sketches and blackboard diagrams to illustrate his lectures. He was also a noted philosopher and I have two of his books on this subject. At that time many of us approached sexual matters with the Victorian middle class attitudes and prejudices about morals, sin, and wickedness in general. So it was a help to have been taught by somebody like Kenneth Walker who could put the facts before us in an interesting and balanced way.

Divorce was rare and not to be mentioned except in hushed voices. Girls could lure men into unwanted marriage if they became pregnant and men were supposed to postpone matrimony until they were established professionally. In my own case I did not think that I would ever enter into a conventional marriage as I thought that asthma and some dependence on anti-asthma drugs would not recommend me to the sort of girl I liked or to her family.

In those days the more adventurous spirits would go to night clubs for entertainment. A friend of mine suggested that I went with him one evening. At the time we were living in the hospital doing midwifery and on that night we were not on call. He led me down some stairs into a basement of a house near Tottenham Court Road and vouched for me to the woman who took our money as we entered.

The atmosphere was hot and stuffy and full of smoke from tobacco. A small but loud band set up a steady and noisy throb accompanied from time to time by strident vocalists. Drinks were being served and the barman would be offered one from time to time. This he would accept with appropriate jolly repartee, take one sip wishing health and good fellowship to all, and put the remainder down out of sight, so that he got paid for one drink several times over. I was a fish out of water in this milieu not knowing how I ought to behave. When a garrulous and potentially amorous blonde came and sat next to me and started to chat me up and want me to supply her with drinks, I lost my nerve and made my escape through the gents' lavatories into the clean air outside. But what astonished me was seeing some of our lecturers enjoying themselves in those surroundings.

Clinical teaching at the bedside was the most important part of a doctor's training and it developed out of the old apprenticeship tradition. As clerks on a 'firm' we had to take the history of the cases allotted to us, examine the patient, carry out simple pathology tests, and be ready to present our findings to our chief before an audience of fellow students and the ward sister, so one was very much put on one's mettle. In the surgical wards we would assist at the dressings of patients where necessary. The experienced ward sisters were often great characters ruling autocratically over medical students and nurses.

Sometimes they would let interested students learn a lot about nursing techniques, and later on when I was working in hospitals as a qualified junior doctor I had occasion to be grateful to them as I could discuss things with the nursing staff from a position of some experience of what their work entailed.

However, the training was limited in some ways by modern standards as consultants had little practical knowledge of general practice which would be the field of work for many of us in the years to come. Many of the patients we saw in the medical wards had chronic or incurable conditions. Rheumatic fever in its various manifestations was common, though it is seldom seen these days.

I clerked on the firm of Dr Alexander Gow an eminent physician who had been present at the battle of Jutland when he was reputed to have reported sick himself after the action with a leaking peptic ulcer. He had a dry sense of humour and would listen carefully as we read out our notes by the bedside and then say 'did you smell the patient?', as he said that acute rheumatic fever patients had a certain foetor. He also made us taste the medicines given to patients and a nurse would join us on the round with a tray of teaspoons.

In those days bottles of medicines containing many ingredients were important parts of treatment. I used to see some patients from the outpatient department swigging their medicines straight from the bottle on the bus going home and paying scant attention to the carefully marked bottles showing half or one teaspoonful to be taken three or four times a day.

Several times a week there would be post-mortem examinations to be attended in 'the temple of truth' as the room was dubbed. Here we learned about the damage diseases could do to various organs and could see how accurate our diagnoses had been. I remember seeing one skull with a depressed fracture caused by a policeman's baton. There had been a drunken riot in which red biddy or methylated spirits had been drunk. The city police had waded in to divide up the crowd and restore order. The pathologist said that the skull was unusually thin and there was not even an inquest.

Midwifery was perhaps the most enjoyable part of the course, and we lived in the hospital to be 'on call'. Most of the deliveries in the wards were uncomplicated, though there were the abnormal and emergency cases dealt with by the consultants and registrars. But, the real fun came when one was 'on district'. By that time I had my own car an open Austin ten two-seater with a dicky. In this I would drive to a house or tenements where I would meet the qualified midwife. Now, for the first time in my life I could see how many people lived around the Angel Islington.

It came as a bit of a shock when I entered a home where the furniture and bed linen had been pawned although there were local government grants to help out if needed. The London cockneys were a tough and cheerful crowd and great survivors. I would arm myself with newspapers of large format like *The Times* to supplement the scanty bedding. Often water was not laid on in individual apartments and one had to go to a shared tap on the staircase landing.

On one occasion I arrived at one such flat before the midwife as I had the use of a car. Things were going wrong, the baby's head had been born with the umbilical cord round the neck stopping it from taking the essential first breaths. I carried some ready sterilised instruments in a fruit preserving jar of my mother's and got ready to cut the cord and relieve the situation. Then all the lights went out and the father who was near hysterics next door had not got the right coins to get the light turned on. Meanwhile in the dark I was trying to find where I had put down my torch. I called for matches and his and my hand met by the door as he handed me the matchbox; by the light of the match I found my torch and the necessary coins, and the rest of the birth posed no problems. So that all was well when the midwife arrived. To have coped with a crisis on one's own successfully was a boost to my medical morale.

On another occasion I had to drive through a busy street market to get at the tenements I was to reach where a birth had started. The barrow boys were not going to let me through easily, until I stood up in my open car and shouted out that Mrs

X. was in labour. Then a way was made for me speedily and the car filled with fruit, vegetables and other goodies for me to give to my patient. All was cockney good humour and cheer.

Stories of adventures on the district abounded. One of my friends arrived to find the father drunk in the bedroom where the birth of his child was imminent. Being a robust chap he took dad by the scruff of the neck and threw him out of the house, after which there was a normal delivery. But the indignant father went to the police claiming that he had been assaulted and ejected from his home. The police arrived and arrested him for being drunk and disorderly. The next day he was in court and fined a sum he could not pay, so was given ten days' detention. The mother and her neighbours thought this was an excellent handling of a difficult clinical situation, and my friend was to find himself quite a hero in the district.

In those days there was a great deal of real poverty about and many of the mothers had a very inadequate diet. In the hospital, doing paediatrics, we saw cases of rickets in children and learned to recognise the clinical signs and X-ray appearances of this disease. There was not much in the way of welfare, but dedicated young priests of high church persuasion would visit our patients and, dressed in black soutanes, would cheer them and bring some light to otherwise drab surroundings.

It was a time when important changes were in the air affecting the British Constitution with events which led up to the resignation of King Edward the Eighth from the throne over his marriage to Mrs Simpson, and also there was the continued rise of Hitler and the Nazis annexing to themselves parts of Europe on various pretexts. Mussolini's invasions of Abyssinia and the horrors of the Spanish Civil War were prominent items of news in the papers. But it was striking how many of the people I met in their homes around the Angel Islington supported King Edward and had his portrait displayed in their rooms.

Oswald Mosley's Blackshirts were also troublesome setting fire to Jewish shops and generally disturbing the peace. One stupid medical student had the temerity to appear in Barts in the Mosley uniform, and was soon dumped into the fountain to cool off. We came to appreciate the cheerfulness and good humour of the people we visited and soon forgot the squalor in which some of them lived.

My father had advised me that should we find ourselves harbouring undesirable livestock in the form of fleas and bugs, a drop of chloroform and a good shake would solve the problem, though I never had occasion to try this myself.

It was Christmas time and once I found myself the guest at a family party of Welsh people around the bedside and cot. That house was spotlessly clean and the family ran a dairy business. Some of the spontaneous Welsh singing in that situation was moving and memorable.

It was interesting to see the city at night and at week-ends when the business people had left. The draymen delivering barrels of beer would pour a pint or so into the mouths of their magnificent horses which would protrude their lower lips to receive their treat and reward for all their patience. In the early hours of the morning the Smithfield meat market would come alive with dealers bargaining. The district was altogether a wonderful way of learning more about human nature and how ordinary people lived.

Then there were the more specialized subjects we had to learn something about, like psychiatry, ear, nose and throat disorders, eyes, and anaesthetics. I had an alarming experience in the latter subject. I was asked to give nitrous oxide, otherwise known as laughing gas, to a large, red-haired, florid lady who needed to have a whitlow on a finger incised. Instead of going under peacefully accompanied by soothing words from me, she suddenly decided that she was on her way to hell: she knelt on the operating table propped up by nurses and students to stop her from falling off and confessed loudly and tearfully to a string of lurid sins from which she sought forgiveness. Nobody had warned me of the difficulties this sort of anaesthesia could give rise to in people who are chronic alcoholics. Practical lessons of this kind are never forgotten.

In psychiatry we were told about the theories of Freud, Adler, and Jung among others, and were taken to see cases at the Royal Bethlehem Hospital.

In those days little was said about the various effects of stress, and many disorders, where there were not ascertainable pathological findings, were labelled as being, in whole or in part, 'functional' meaning something like being of poor moral fibre or not controlling one's emotions enough to want to cope with life's vagaries and problems. From the treatment point of view such a label meant that little or nothing could be done to help the patient. In those days there were many large psychiatric hospitals where many patients spent most of their lives as chronic institutional inmates with little treatment available to help restore them to some sort of life in the outside community. Fortunately, there have been great advances in treatment and understanding of mental disorders.

There were visits to a fever hospital in the East End of London, and we used to travel there by car, myself driving my Austin ten two-seater with two passengers in the dicky seat if the weather was fine. Sometimes another car load of students would try to pelt us with rotten tomatoes to which we would reply by waiting in ambush in side roads. This dangerous game finished when a tomato whizzed across me sitting innocently in a traffic jam in the Commercial Road East to hit a lorry driver in the next lane to me. I, being innocent, was quick to sympathize with him as the other car made its get-away.

In the fever hospital we saw distressing cases of diphtheria, some with unpleasant complications. In those days vaccination against this infection was far from being universal and it was a fairly common disease.

The international situation was getting tense leading up to the Munich crisis, and friends of mine in the Territorial Army were getting themselves into a state of readiness for war. Communism had been popular among some *avant-garde* intellectual students and there had been an attempt to send fraternal greetings to Moscow from the Students Union. Those of us more traditionally minded had managed to rustle up some opposition to this idea and it was turned down at a rowdy meeting. Some of the more vehement reds of that time went on to have distinguished medical careers and were to serve in the forces as medical officers and good patriots.

We were coming to the end of our clinical course and were swatting for our qualifying examinations hoping to be doctors before war should break out. We were given some alarming lectures on what to expect if and when that should happen. On a hot summer's day in 1939 we assembled to learn about what might be expected of us in an air-raid. An unfortunate porter was dressed up in gas-proof clothing and wore a gasmask to cover his face. No skin was exposed as mustard gas was expected. This outfit was too much for the porter who soon slumped to the floor in a fainting attack and he had to be rescued from anti-gas gear.

During these years just before the war I was living with my parents and sisters in a house in Addison Road in Kensington. Having my own small car was a great advantage to me as it enabled me to enjoy my freedom. Asthma, as usual, made strenuous team games impossible, but with suitable precautions such as taking ephedrine tablets I could enjoy such things as horse riding, beagling, and sometimes tennis or squash when I could stop or go slow if necessary. In those years inhalation treatment started to become available and a hand-worked rubber bulb blew air into an inhaler through a solution of appropriate drugs. This meant that incipient attacks could be controlled more easily, and if necessary, privately by retreating into a lavatory.

Having a car I used to go horse riding on Wimbledon Common and in Richmond Park, often before breakfast in the summer and at that early hour there was a pleasant and informal camaraderie among the horsemen who were from many walks of life, retired military officers, police, rangers, and others including humble students like myself. To improve my skills I had some lessons at the school of equitation at Richmond where the instructors were ex-cavalry men from the army school of riding at Weedon.

On some Sundays I would drive to Storrington in Sussex and enjoy exhilarating canters and gallops across the South Downs, often accompanied by the Borzoi hound owned by the stables where we hired the horses. After the ride we would enjoy a good lunch at a pub and then return to London for the next week's work feeling very happy with life.

One summer I went on a short riding holiday near Wimborne on a course run by the owners of the Wimbledon stables where I usually hired my mounts. I also had the chances on other holidays of exploring the Quantocks, Exmoor and Dartmoor on horseback. The lady who owned the horses on Dartmoor claimed that she had gypsy blood in her and that she had the gift of second sight and had visual perceptions of past events concerning the history of Dartmoor from far back in time. The going there could be rough and the horses were equipped with coiled rope halters so that in theory, should they sink into a bog, the rider would leap off onto firm land and pull them out. Fortunately, I never had to try this manoeuvre.

I used to go beagling with a pack which was privately owned by a group of people including friends of mine who were students at the Royal Veterinary College. We used to hunt over parts of the Hertfordshire countryside near to Cockfosters. Hares tend to run in circles so that all I had to do if I started to get exercise asthma was to stay still until my medicaments had worked, by which time the hunt would have come close to where I was. For a short period I was a member of the Budokwai judo club near Victoria station, though I never took it seriously enough to get very far with it.

All in all it was a good period in life despite the anxieties coming from the international situation, and on the personal level, anxieties about passing examinations and beginning a professional career.

I was not ready for the Cambridge University final M.B. which I would finish at Christmas 1939, so I entered myself for the Conjoint Board finals in June 1939 hoping for an earlier qualification even if it was considered to be inferior to a university M.B. I managed to pass and was congratulating myself on having become a proper doctor, when I was presented with a bill for forty pounds to pay for the preliminary examinations from which I had been exempted as I had the second M.B. This, on top of the entry fees, was too much for me to pay out of my father's allowances to me. So after attending the impressive ceremony which the Royal College of Surgeons gave to welcome its new members I went to a telephone call box to tell my father the news and ask for what in those days was a substantial sum of money.

I had not told my parents that I was taking the examination as I dreaded the post mortem questions which my mother would ask on such occasions as she was ever anxious that we should come up to expectations. My father thought that I was pulling his leg, but was delighted when he knew it to be true. Soon afterwards, I was brought down to earth again when a friend of his, in his and my presence, asked me 'when would I be starting to walk the wards as a student?'

War was now almost inevitable in the near future, though we continued to hope for some miracle whereby it could be avoided. For myself I was greatly relieved to know that I could be of use in a crisis as a qualified doctor and would probably serve in London where my family were living.

Chapter 5

Young Doctor

It is the ambition of most young doctors to work in a junior capacity on one of the 'firms' on which he had trained: this would be the first step on the ladder for those with ambitions to become consultants in future days. I was told quietly, though I have forgotten by whom, that it might be a good idea for me to join a medical Freemasons' Lodge. I shrugged off this suggestion without much thought as the idea of a secret male society with elaborate and complex rituals which did not mean anything to me, was frightening to someone of my temperament. It made me wonder how much nepotism counted even in a medical career. However, I became a junior in the outpatient department. My chief, with a solemn expression, said to me 'my boy remember that big fleas have little fleas and so ad infinitum. You are the littlest flea in this circus so don't worry if you are asked to carry the blame.' I still had part of the final Cambridge M.B. to complete and hoped to sit this examination about Christmas 1939.

Meanwhile, I was due for a holiday. I had had ambitious plans to ride over parts of Hungary with a pack horse to carry the luggage. I was going with an old preparatory school friend now in the regular army. His leave was cancelled owing to the menacing international situation, so I had to change my plans.

My mother and my two sisters with a friend had gone to Bergun in the Engadine in Switzerland on my recommendation. With two student friends I had enjoyed a skiing holiday there earlier in the year. I decided to join them at the Hotel Weisses Kreux and took a ticket to Bergun at Victoria Station. To be back in a small alpine village in a friendly hotel was just what I needed physically and spiritually. We went for long walks in the foothills of the mountains and took day trips to places like Pontresina and St. Moritz by train. For the time we forgot about Herr Hitler and enjoyed the company of two German families in the hotel. In her young days my mother had been a music student in Germany and got on well with the people.

However, the war clouds seemed to be gathering and I rang up the British Consul to see whether we should return to England. He said that he had had no official advice to suggest this to tourists like ourselves. On the next day the travel agents my mother had used rang to say that they were arranging a special train back to the channel ports for their customers. I, travelling on an ordinary ticket, decided to stay on a day or two on my own, as we had got a bit blasé about crisis news. So, I made up m mind to cross over a pass above the Morterasch Glacier to come down to St. Moritz the other side and then catch the train back to Bergun.

It was a lovely day, with flowers out in the alpine meadows, and the Swiss cows grazing contentedly to the sound of their cowbells; the views were superb with a backdrop of high snow-covered mountains and glaciers. Near the top of the pass I joined a young man of about my age, also on his own, and started to chat with him. I found he was a German. Inevitably, we asked each other about the situation in Europe. He said that Hitler was about to invade Poland, so I asked him why he had not been called up. He said that he was on a hut to hut tour and so no telegram was likely to reach him. So we went up to the restaurant at the top of the pass together, and had some drinks and food. When the time came to part we wrung each other's hands and wished each other personal luck in the coming conflict hoping that we could meet again in happier times. That evening when I returned to the hotel, I found the proprietor and the chef preparing to go into the mountain passes with the arms they kept ready for mobilization to defend the Swiss frontiers.

Basle station where the frontiers of Switzerland, France and Germany meet was blacked out and there was a general air of tension in the crowds of people waiting for trains to take them home. I was lucky, and pushing some money into the hands of a sleeping car attendant through a window, I managed to get a sleeper. The route to Ostend was close to the frontier of France and Germany, and we were frequently put into sidings while troop trains were busy along the Maginot line.

When we arrived at Ostend the day was sunny and hot, and there were no ferry boats to take across the channel for some hours. I spent the time bathing and enjoying the beach while hearing some bizarre stories and rumours from other travellers from distant parts of Europe.

Eventually we boarded a crowded boat, but the weather remained fine and calm. Once or twice a destroyer came and circled us, and there was a Sunderland flying boat about at one time. The atmosphere was one of unreality and tension. Eventually, I reached home to the relief of my parents. I had had a comfortable journey myself thanks to the sleeper, but my unfortunate mother and sisters had had little sleep or rest in the crowded special train organized by the travel agency.

London was getting ready for war with air raid shelters being cleaned out and then equipped with rugs and candles; important buildings were being protected by sandbags, and blackout measures were being checked. Perhaps the sight that struck me most was seeing some of the Horse Guards putting their magnificent mounts onto trains to take them to France. As a small boy I had accepted the sight of the Life Guards and the Blues with wonder and pleasure as they played their parts in so many ceremonial occasions.

Now, instead of gorgeous uniforms, the men were in khaki with tin helmets and gasmasks at the ready. It filled me with horror to think what these men and their beautiful horses might have to face very soon, and I had seen many pictures of the First World War. Also my ageing parents would, this time, be in

a target area as they had no thought of leaving London, and my
father was doing some industrial medical work.

I, myself, was a casualty doctor at St Bartholomew's Hospital
waiting for the air raids to start. Most departments of the
hospital had been evacuated to safer areas such as St. Albans.
Operating theatres had been prepared below ground level and
the ground floors were heavily protected by sandbags. As
things turned out, this became the period of the so-called
phoney war, and I had plenty of time to study for the last bit of
my Cambridge M.B. But I was getting restless and wanted to get
on with my medical apprenticeship. I applied for and got a job
as a house physician at the Corbett Hospital at Stourbridge in
the Midlands. Although my father was disappointed that I
would not wait for any opening to appear at Barts., I could
look forward to a busy life in general medicine under a consultant from the Birmingham teaching hospital group.

I went up for the interview and stayed the previous night in
the Grand Hotel in Birmingham. I groped my way in the
blackout to the old Theatre Royal in New Street where the
comedian Richard Hearn was performing in a variety programme. He made me laugh and forget my many doubts at this
difficult time. As a result the interview was encouraging and I
accepted a job which carried a lot of responsibility and which
would give me more general experience than one might get
under some London consultants specialising in somewhat narrow fields.

The Corbett Hospital was then a small hospital standing in
extensive grounds with a small lake and wooded areas. The
resident staff consisted of a Resident Surgical Officer and several of us juniors of varying experience. If we got into difficult
problems we could, in theory, ring our chiefs in Birmingham,
but they could be reluctant to come to our aid in the blackout.
Some of the local practitioners who had worked with our chiefs
in Birmingham would be available when help was needed.

The work was fascinating but very demanding. Soon we had
to deal with an outbreak of meningitis without having the
antibiotics now available. As the winter went by things became

more difficult as some doctors and other staff joined the forces and were not replaced.

My chief job was that of house physician, but I was also house surgeon to the Eye Department run by a young lady ophthalmologist recently graduated into the consultant position. I did my share of emergency casualty work, and gave anaesthetics at emergency operations. Judged by modern standards I was doing work much beyond what I should have been called upon to do with my limited experience. Then the pathologist went off to the war and I got asked from time to time to do post-mortem examinations.

Lastly, I was put in charge of the dispensary which meant keeping an eye on stocks. I found to my dismay that drawers containing drugs had been tampered with, and by sticking bits of black cotton across the key holes I knew that things had been taken and not recorded. The guilty person was a young house officer, and I had to tell the administrator that I could not be responsible any more for keeping drug records.

Lastly, I was asked to lecture to the nurses in the nurses' home, which in those days was very much a female preserve. So I would go over with an escort of the sister tutor who kept a firm eye on me, and took notes of everything I said. Inevitably the cheekier of the young girls would attempt to upset me by asking awkward or silly questions. It was usually possible to trap them by asking them seemingly simple questions which they could not easily answer. It was all good natured fun even if the sister tutor frowned on any levity.

Stourbridge is in the black country with heavy metal-working industries and also glass cutting; a canal system ran through it. I got to like the people who were great characters although I had to get used to their accents and idioms of speech. I was able to visit some of the factories including an iron works where I learned what iron puddling meant, working near to hot furnaces and handling heavy weights of molten metal. To compensate for sweating the men would drink quantities of a light beer. Once, where a large steam driven hammer was at work amid great clamour and sparks flying everywhere, there was a sudden lull and the local character responsible for the din descended from his control box to give us his rendering of bird songs. The glass cutting factories were always interesting, and I still have a mug with cuttings and engraving done by various artists in the works.

For recreation there was riding over the Clent hills and bicycle rides to the Severn Valley and beyond. Through relations I had some introductions to some pleasant and interesting families living near the Clent hills, and others at Stourport on Severn. The winter was cold and I had my skates and my skis with me so enjoyed some mild winter sports. The skis enabled me to get to a farm cut off by drifts.

I have happy memories of the Corbett Hospital and a few years ago I had the opportunity of returning there to give a lecture. It had changed into a much bigger hospital with new buildings and all the adjuncts necessary to modern medicine. The old wards where I had cut my medical teeth were lost in these new buildings. But my day was made when a lady introduced herself to me: she had been one of the pharmacists and had come out of retirement specially to meet me again.

When my six months was over, I was again faced by the problem of what I should do next. It was obvious that the war would become more violent as the traditional campaigning season had approached. I thought that some surgical experience would be useful and I applied for a job at Selly Oak Hospital in Birmingham as a house surgeon. I was to be paid at the rate of £350 a year instead of £110 a year I had been getting at the Corbett Hospital. Selly Oak paid more as it was run by the Council and not just by charitable donations as was the common practice before the National Health Service.

Most of my friends were joining the services, but being uncertain about my health I thought I would be more useful, at any rate for the present, in civilian medicine. Everyone thought there would be devastating air raids and this reassured me that I was not running away from an ordeal for which my friends had volunteered so eagerly. Soon Dunkirk was upon us and there was a very real threat of a German invasion. I was indeed fortunate in being a qualified doctor able to work in a hospital.

The collapse of Europe under the weight of Hitler's *blitzkrieg* brought with it a sense of urgent reality. No longer were any of us able to live in a fantasy world of relative security: invasion and the iron heel were not now just remote possibilities. The miracle of Dunkirk with the survival of the core of the British army was followed by the resolute speeches of Winston Churchill, who made each of us aware of being caught up in something bigger than our own individual destinies: this was a heady feeling.

The sense of belonging to something much greater than one's own personal self was strong. This was the old urge to self transcendence which can lead men to glory or to folly. We felt that all our culture, our traditions, and our freedom to follow our own stars within our limits were threatened, and that should we lose the war to Hitler we might become slaves physically and mentally in a life without much meaning, purpose or value.

Meanwhile self transcendence in Germany meant the uncritical dedication to a fantasy world of domination and brutality by a self-styled master race. The old problem of the maintenance of the individual's personal integrity and critical faculties when strong group emotions are aroused is one which history has shown to have eluded understanding by the mass of humanity.

Selly Oak Hospital is a large hospital serving a big population working in local industries. Besides routine medical and surgical duties it undertook a large amount of casualty work especially as a municipal welfare officer known as the relieving officer could demand admissions of cases even if it meant putting up extra beds in the centre of the wards: this was done quite often. The consultants were whole time physicians and surgeons without private practices. They were skilled, hardworking and dedicated men and women. Normally, they would have had as juniors much more experienced doctors than I was, but so many had been called up for military service that they were becoming a scarcity. There were three surgical firms and three medical ones and an obstetric and gynaecological firm. Duty rosters were arranged so that a surgical team was ready for any air-raid casualties with one in reserve: a third team would be resting.

Besides the routine acute work there was a part of the hospital given over to chronic cases and to those with incurable conditions. Each junior medical officer was allocated a ward in this block. Many of the cases in these wards were very distressing as patients were crowded by modern standards, and nursing and physiotherapy services were limited. Despite many difficulties, the middle aged nursing sister in charge of the ward allotted to me did devoted work with few resources and a minimal staff of people to help her.

The firm I worked in was headed by Mr. Philip Reading who, besides being a general surgeon, was also the Ear, Nose and Throat consultant. A man of short stature, he had a quick brain able to penetrate to the core of the many clinical problems and to resolve them speedily. As an operator he had nimble and accurate fingers in the true craftsman's traditions of his speciality. He taught me a lot and in time let me do routine operations to remove tonsils and adenoids. I enjoyed doing these operations if I had a good anaesthetist who could get the right depth of anaesthesia: too deep and the patient's recovery would be longer than was wanted: too shallow and the throat reflexes would make the operation impossible.

There were many cases of infected mastoids, and these patients needed complex operations to remove dead bone, and afterwards they had to endure repeated unpleasant dressings. The advent of antibiotics have made these chronic mastoid infections rare and I saw few if any in my years in general practice after the war.

Then the air raids started. The Midlands with all its heavy and light industries was an obvious target, though it did not suffer on the scale that London did in the blitz, except for the Coventry raid when the old cathedral was destroyed. There was an air raid siren located in the hospital worked by a porter who was also an air raid warden. Once, in daylight, German bomb-ers came over, evidently trying to destroy the Longbridge motor factory, then making aircraft. The warning wail went off, but many of us were overcome by curiosity and looked into the skies. Eventually, but too late, a squadron of our fighters appeared: the enemy had dropped some bombs with little damage. A certain amount of anti-aircraft flak was flying about and a bit hit the siren operator on the nose causing him to pull the all clear lever by accident at the height of the activity.

The night raids were more serious, and on some nights we were kept busy dealing with casualties: these included old people, children and cripples, besides the normally healthier section of the population. Comparatively inexperienced as I was, I found myself operating on limbs which sometimes needed amputation, and dealing with eye injuries as I had done some eye work at the Corbett Hospital and there was no regular eye department at Selly Oak.

On one occasion I went into the operating theatre at about six o'clock one evening to assist with the normal emergency cases: as we were finishing a raid started, and the casualties began to come in. We were kept busy until next morning when the relief surgical team took over. Just as I was getting to sleep a delayed action bomb went off in the hospital grounds injur-ing men of a bomb disposal unit trying to deal with it.

A very heavy load was carried by the consultants who would deal with injuries to the head, chest and abdomen requiring their experience and expertise. All at the hospital worked hard as a team with no thought of their own fatigue under the efficient leadership of Mr. Hugh Carson the superintendent who was also a surgeon.

After six months I was due for a holiday, and I was able to meet my mother at Moreton-in-the-Marsh for a few days in a hotel. Unfortunately there were some well-to-do refugees from the Midland cities taking refuge there, and on finding that I was a doctor they started to discuss their manifold minor ailments in the public rooms, to my discomfort. This became too much, and I said out loud that I would give them a consultation in private if they paid me twenty-five pounds in advance. My mother thought this very rude of me, as it probably was, but it had the desired effect and we could enjoy the rest of our holiday and do some motoring on saved up petrol coupons, of which we had accumulated a supply as my father did not drive and my sisters were on war work.

By this time I was interested in surgery and wanted to get more experience, so I applied for a post at York where I thought I would get more time to catch up on my reading. For various reasons this job was unsatisfactory, and the elderly surgeon I worked for left me too much responsibility without teaching me much. Always, I was haunted by the question as to whether I should try to join one of the services as virtually all my medical contemporaries had done. I felt I was missing out on the main experience of my age, and once more would feel that physical disability was isolating me.

So I gave notice, having somehow been introduced to the medical director of The Retreat, a famous mental hospital founded by the Quaker family Tuke. I think that this came about because some old Quaker friends of my family, Dr. and Mrs. Phear, had mentioned my name to Dr. Poole, the director of the Retreat. He engaged me on a locum basis to fill in time before I returned to London to be casualty officer at the North Middlesex Hospital.

I had felt a bit guilty at being in York while my parents in London were in constant danger from air raids. My father had refused to leave London and was kept busy at industrial medicine, a subject in which he had always been interested. Both my parents bore the raids with great courage and endurance. In one letter I had they said that two fire bombs had fallen near the house, and though my father had put his out first, my mother said that she had extinguished hers better because she had followed the A.R.P. instructions to the letter. At the North Middlesex I would be in London and in some sense able to share with them whatever horrors Hitler had in store for us.

As things turned out the weeks I spent as a resident doctor at The Retreat were to be a very happy and lucky break for me. I had learned little about mental health as a student, and now I had the opportunity to work in the leading private mental hospital in the country. I was also fortunate in having Dr. Poole as the medical director. He taught me a lot and would show me how to listen and learn from the patients. For instance, I would play billiards with a chronic alcoholic who had spent a life in billiard saloons and who knew a lot about the game, but his chronic alcoholism made his hands shaky so that I could usually keep up with him. The doctor patient relationship would be in abeyance and I got some inkling of the workings of his mind.

There were many difficult and tragic cases needing treatment or close supervision. A few patients were having treatment with insulin to the stage of coma, and they required skilled attention: also there were one or two having electric convulsion therapy which was new to me and which at that time seemed to be a drastic therapy, though later it was to become a fairly common sort of treatment for some kinds of depression.

In those days the word 'stress' was seldom if ever used as being a factor in mental illness, but one very disturbed young woman who was on insulin treatment had had some unpleasant experiences in escaping from France, and she had seen a refugee ship bombed and sunk. She made a very good recovery and such cases were very rewarding to the staff of the hospital.

On some nights there would be raids on the R.A.F. bomber airfields in Yorkshire and we would have to take the patients down to the basement where it was supposed they would be safer. This meant that depressives and those with manic tendencies would be together, the former moaning about 'why should it happen to them' and 'the cruelty of fate', while some of the latter would play act or squabble, but on the whole enjoy all the fuss.

There was also humour, as when in the course of a Sunday service in the chapel a lady got up and declaimed 'the Lord provideth meat thou wist not of', as she produced a string of sausages from the bag she was carrying. Perhaps the miracle was apt in those days of strict rationing. Another patient reading a lesson was so carried away that he would not stop and had to be led gently back to his pew.

Some of the patients had impressive mental and physical skills, but for one reason or another were unable to adapt to living in the outside world. There were several doctors needing treatment, and there were writers, one of whom carried on a very academic correspondence about the poet Ossian, and was able to compose verse in the idiom of that author. A calculating genius was challenged by Dr. Poole to say how many hours there would be in the next nine years or so. His answers came quickly, but did not match our lengthy calculations with pencil and paper, but he pointed out that it was we who had forgotten to take the leap years into account.

An artist suffering from general paralysis of the insane – a syphilitic complication – painted some exciting surrealist pictures. He was treated by being given malaria to give him episodes of fever. That was a common treatment in those days, and an infected mosquito was sent up from a laboratory in a sort of match box covered with a mesh, and this was strapped to his thigh. He improved rapidly, and as he did so his art changed into paintings of York in the pictorial tradition of the pictures on sale in the tourist shops.

The grounds of The Retreat were extensive and beautiful. At the time of the Civil War armies had fought around there and cannon balls had been found in the grounds.

The Quaker motto 'the caring of friends gives proof of humanity' set the tone of the place and the atmosphere was relaxed and friendly, besides being of high professional standard from the point of view of treatment and caring. This came out well at the staff conferences where I learned a lot about this aspect of medicine. Even if that elusive factor 'the person' could become buried under the manifestations of a breakdown in mental integration, the core of individuality remained. I learned a new respect for the wonders of the human brain which was to be of great value to me later on in general practice and as an industrial doctor.

As in all branches of medicine, many advances are being made in psychiatry, and practical experience for me had begun to supersede the rather dull theoretical instruction we had been given as students on such topics as the writings of Freud, Adler, and Jung. I was really sorry to leave The Retreat to take up my post as Casualty Officer at the North Middlesex Hospital in London. It was a busy and responsible job, but my evenings were usually free and I had wanted to catch up on my medical reading.

I borrowed my parents' car to drive to the North Middlesex Hospital with my gear, but ran out of petrol when taking it home and had to park it at a garage until I had collected some petrol coupons to enable me to complete the journey. Then misfortune struck, and I developed acute appendicitis and had to be operated on the same evening after I had spent some hours assisting at operations on casualties. While I was under the anaesthetic there was quite a sharp air raid with about thirty casualties being brought into the hospital, and I only learned about this the next morning.

At this stage of the war the threats of invasion had receded, and most of the action was taking place in North Africa and at sea. I took the plunge and volunteered for the R.A.F. as a doctor. I had expected to be made C3, but fit for home duties. With the aid of ephedrine tablets and the use of inhalation therapy I had reasonable control of my asthma, and I had managed to work for long hours in some onerous posts. Also, by this time I was practised at the arts of guile and dissimulation to hide my weakness. I had a somewhat cursory medical examination at an Air Ministry centre in London and was passed as being fit.

As a casualty officer I saw a vast variety of medical and surgical cases ranging from the trivial to the serious, and had to make quick decisions about how they should be handled. Fortunately, I had an excellent experienced staff nurse to help me. She was a very pretty girl with an Irish brogue and a sharp temper mitigated by a ready sense of humour. Soon after I left the hospital I heard that she had been killed in an air raid when part of a hospital had been hit.

Leaving the North Middlesex Hospital meant the end of another chapter in my life. The job had involved more responsibility as regards decision making than had previous posts, but again I had enjoyed the work.

For recreation I had been able to spend some hours on the farm where my sister was working in the land army, and I found that turning hay with a horse drawn hay rake was good relaxation as I sat behind the rump of a willing horse which knew the job better than I did. I also hand milked cows which I did not find so easy or pleasant, though they were amiable enough. Sometimes I would go riding on a hired horse through Epping Forest which in those times was not overcrowded and there were some pleasant pubs in the area frequented by other horsemen. One night after a raid I feared for the stables from where I hired my horse, but heard that all was well and that, surprisingly, the horses had remained calm. Domesticated animals are good antidotes to the problems created by human aberrations.

Chapter 6

R.A.F. (Part 1)

By early 1941 all my contemporaries who had shared my student years with me at Cambridge and St. Barts Hospital were in the services leaving civilian medicine to those who were reserved for one reason or another or who were deemed to be medically unfit. The inner pressures to conform and to join one of the services were strong. By this time I had gained more self confidence than I had ever had before: I had found that I could work long hours and could cope with the stresses and uncertainties of hospital life in wartime. I knew that with my asthmatic tendencies army life was not for me and there was a long waiting list for the navy, but I thought I might apply for the R.A.F.V.R. where I might be accepted even in a restricted medical category for home service, as life on an airfield would be unlikely to be more demanding than it could be in civilian hospitals.

Aeroplanes had had a fascination for me as a boy and my father had taken me to the annual R.A.F. displays at Hendon which we both had enjoyed greatly. My father had also taken me for a flight over London in one of Imperial Airways' splendid four-engined biplanes based at Croyden aerodrome. He sat bolt upright wearing a bowler hat, one hand clutching a rolled umbrella and the other hand the table in front of him. It was a great adventure for both of us.

The day came when the official envelope arrived ordering me to attend for a medical examination at one of the Air Ministry buildings in London. We were told to strip and dress ourselves in a coarse, R.A.F. dressing gown and were then kept waiting for what seemed hours before facing the ordeal of the examination which was very official, correct and cold. Some felt humiliated by the off-hand and unwelcoming atmosphere, though experience of public school made this easy for me to cope with, but my exasperation rose as time went by because I had tickets for the opera and had arranged to take out my current girl friend.

No objection was made to my asthmatic history, and I was not wheezing as I had taken an ephedrine tablet shortly before. I was told curtly to await further instructions and that I could expect to be called up in a matter of a few weeks. So, I was faced with a period of anxious waiting, and asked myself whether I should have made more of my asthmatic history and opted out of service life.

When the call-up notice came I was given a time and date to report to the medical officers training centre at Harrogate. Before then a uniform had to be ordered and the basic kit collected.

My father was the medical officer to the Army and Navy Stores in London and they had a long tradition of supplying the needs of officers in the various services of the British Empire. The head of the tailoring department was an old friend, though a rather awesome figure always immaculately dressed in a tail coat, striped trousers, gleaming top hat, and cravat with jewelled pin. With his ample figure and rubicund face this all made him an imposing person. So I started off properly dressed and kitted as a Flying Officer with the good wishes of my old friend.

It turned out that others were not so fortunate: one had had his uniform made by the village tailor who had sewn the broad stripe of an Air Commodore on his sleeves as he thought it looked more impressive. This it did as we embryo R.A.F.V.R. medicos received some very smart salutes from other ranks as we gathered at King's Cross railway station and we were uncertain whether we should all acknowledge the salutes or just the supposed Air Commodore. Soon we were in the train to Harrogate armed with our first class rail passes.

Harrogate was a cold and raw place in November, but we were reasonably comfortably billeted in what had once been a good class hotel. Once more I was faced with all the feelings of uncertainty of being a new boy, though by now I had acquired a lot of experience of being a raw junior having to find his feet in a novel situation. Nothing had been so bad as being a new boy at my public school and I was more at ease than some of my fellows who had not had that experience.

We were to have one week in which to become officers and gentlemen as the saying used to go. We rose early in the morning and soon after daylight we had drill under the direction of a Sergeant who was our shepherd for the week. The drill was fun for those of us who had been in a school O.T.C. as we knew the basic exercises and where to put our feet at the various words of command. Those who had not had this training would get confused, and this was so with a surgeon who, entering the service as a specialist, had the two rings of a Flight Lieutenant as opposed to our single rings. We took it in turns to command the squad and I am afraid that we tried our best to get his feet tied up with difficult orders.

Our Sergeant was a good hearted man with a sense of humour. Once when passing a pretty girl on her way to work the medico in charge that day ordered an 'eyes right' and the embarrassed young lady found herself being saluted by the squad of medical officers. 'This is not the proper occasion for general salute, sirs', shouted our Sergeant with a broad grin on his face. He was always punctilious about ending any order or request with the word 'sir'. At the end of the week we gave him a party.

The lectures were a mixed bag. Those on service etiquette and customs designed for peacetime seemed to be a long way from the realities of war, and many of us had seen bomb casualties in our civilian work. We were told that on being posted to a new station we should call on the Commanding Officer armed with two visiting cards, one for him and one for his wife. Saluting, we were informed, derived from ancient days when knights in armour would raise their visors on meeting each other to show friendly intentions. It took two lectures to explain the procedures and forms to be used if an airman should lose or break his spectacles.

I still have the R.A.F. pocket book of 1937. This contains a mass of detailed information on many topics including such matters as butchering and what to do if one is involved in a forced landing in the desert and how to approach and treat the Bedouins one goes to for help. For instance, one should leave one's dog tied in the aircraft.

But a sense of reality and urgency returned when we were addressed by a flying personnel medical officer who was a qualified pilot and who had flown in a Spitfire in combat sweeps across the channel. He gave us our first real insight into what life was like on an operational station and the stresses borne by the aircrew. Being, as we were, essentially non combatants he told us what we could do to aid and succour the fighting men.

The week passed all too quickly and soon we were to be faced with the lottery of a first posting and facing yet again the 'new boy' anxieties. We had formed friendships and learned a lot about service life and about ourselves and our inadequacies in coping with it. One of our colleagues was a large Polish doctor who had had hair raising experiences in escaping from Europe into allied territory. In the duller lectures he would doze off and when roused sharply by an indignant lecturer would plead ignorance of the English language which in reality he could understand quite well.

When the posting notices came I was somewhat dismayed to find that I was to go to the R.A.F. Airman Recruiting Centre at Blackpool. Once again I said farewell to friends I had got to know and like, and set off alone on a railway journey which was to involve delays and changes of trains. When I arrived at Blackpool it was raining and dark in the late evening with the strict blackout. Eventually, I managed to get a taxi and asked to be taken to the R.A.F. headquarters.

It appeared that there were several R.A.F. administrative headquarters in the town and I asked to be taken to the nearest one. I got out of the cab, said goodnight to the driver and went with my gear up a path to the door.

Here I was challenged by a sentry with a loaded rifle – as I supposed it to be – and was confronted by him with the fixed bayonet pointing at my alarmed body. I was asked to give the password which of course I did not know. I soon realised that the sentry was as scared as I was and that he too was a new recruit trying to obey orders. I sympathized with his lot and promised to stand still in the rain until he had found an N.C.O. I did not feel that I had made a very good start at being an officer.

Blackpool was one of the big initial training centres for airmen entering the service as volunteers or conscripts, and possibly it was the only one. It was also a centre for the B.B.C. and there were many entertainers both in and out of uniform in reserved jobs keeping up the spirits of the country by performing on the air.

We had sick parades in a large church hall requisitioned for the purpose. There were standard pills and potions for the majority of ailments with which we had to deal including the famous number 9 for constipation. Those who were too ill to go on sick parade were seen in their billets which were generally in the erstwhile holiday lodging houses. I would do rounds accompanied by a medical N.C.O. or a medical orderly equipped with the remedies. Medically, the work was boring when compared with what I had become used to in hospitals. The age range was limited with no children or old people or chronic cases to see.

There was plenty of form filling, routine inoculations and inspections to be done, and I began to feel that I had made the wrong decision in joining up. Also, Blackpool, in a chilly November with rain storms sweeping in from the Irish Sea, was unappealing and very different to the jolly, highly illuminated holiday resort one had heard about before the war when its piers and famous bars had brightened up the lives of so many holiday makers from grim industrial towns in the north. Now, even the foreshore was littered with anti-tank defences.

However, I managed to hire a horse and when possible rode it along the shore between the defences. This made me feel better and it was an escape from the officers' mess where I met few people I found congenial. Less dull were some of the medical other ranks, some of whom had led interesting lives in peacetime. One was a jockey by trade, and he had with him a gold watch given by a grateful racehorse owner who had employed him. He told me that he had collected several more gold watches in his career. Then there were the part time entertainers and radio comics who were medical orderlies in daytime.

Fortunately, after a few weeks a posting came through for me, and I was ordered to report to the aircrew receiving centre in London (A.C.R.C.). Here those who had volunteered for aircrew duties went through the processes of initial training and drill besides having further medical examinations and assessment of their education levels. Psychologically, they were given personality tests to see whether they were best suited for particular duties.

For instance, fighter pilots needed quick reactions and re-flexes while bomber pilots had to have the ability to concentrate on their instruments and to gain the confidence of their crews. Professor Bartlett from Cambridge University had devised some complex and interesting tests to enable this grading to be done effectively.

Medically, all recruits went through a Mass Radiography examination to eliminate any undetected tuberculosis or other lung disease. In those days Mass Radiography was in its pioneer stages. The men were billeted in luxury flats around Regent's Park with one block housing the administrative and medical centre. I was given permission to live at home with my parents in Kensington and I used a push bicycle as transport even in the blackout when headlamps had to be shaded. On some nights I had to remain on duty for emergencies including air raids.

To begin with I was given dull routine work including help-ing with mass inoculations and vaccinations. Perhaps the most tedious job of all was doing F.F.I. (freedom from infection) inspections. On one occasion I was doing this at Lord's cricket ground. Each man would have to drop his trousers as he stood in front of me so that I might detect any body lice lurking on him. As one pair of trousered legs came before me, I asked angrily why he was still clothed, to find that I was inadvertently addressing a distinguished member of Lord's and had failed to recognise his face.

For a time I was Adjutant to the Senior Medical Officer whom I had not taken to as I found him to be ambitious and arrogant. The Commanding Officer was a well known cricketer, and a pleasant man with a difficult job. One of the senior officers had become a millionaire as a pioneer of greyhound racing and there was a certain amount of nepotism in the senior ranks. My spell as an Adjutant soon came to an end much to my relief as I had put up one or two blacks in dealing with dull paper work including telling the truth when I wrote 'I dont know why' in the space reserved for stating 'the reason for forwarding the documents' which in that case seemed to be senseless.

I was then put in charge of testing the cadets for their night vision capacity. This move, though at first unpromising, was to turn out to be a lucky break for me. As the war dragged on more and more flying was done at night both in Bomber Command and in Fighter Command where new techniques of intercepting enemy bombers with fighters directed onto their targets by radar were being rapidly developed. Other com-mands were also to need night flying and the Royal Navy, too, was adopting R.A.F. selection and training methods.

A typical operation report derived from one night-fighter goes something like this. 'Directed onto a target getting a visual at 2,500 feet range: Identified as Heinkel 111. Got to within 80 yds. of the He and 20–30 yds. beneath. Opened fire: immediate white flash in the fuselage central section and pieces flew off. Enemy aircraft went into a vertical dive. Half a minute later the sky all round me was lit up by an enormous orange flash and glow. Bits of the enemy aircraft were seen to be burning on the ground.'

In 1942 the Germans were advancing rapidly into Russia, and if they had been successful in destroying the Russian army, they would have switched the bulk of their formidable bomber force to raid this country. Hence there was considerable urgency for the development of defences and for the training of aircrew in the use of sophisticated aircraft and technology.

Then as the German war effort began to falter, and as more Mosquito aircraft became operational, attention was given to night intruder raids on selected sensitive targets in occupied Europe. This required an understanding of the effects of moonlight on buildings, roads, railways and water. The night vision schools did what they could to give ground simulation training, and practical training in Anson communication planes adapted as flying classrooms.

At this point it is worth saying briefly what are the reasons for testing for night vision capacity. Essentially the eye can be likened to a miniature camera with a zoom lens. In daylight the object being viewed is focused on an area of the retina at the back of the eye where light and colour sensitive cone cells are concentrated in an area called the macula which is capable of high resolution permitting the perception of detail. At six to ten degrees off are found the rod cells which are insensitive to colour while being sensitive to contrast of light and shade. In the dark they accumulate a pigment called rhodopsin which will render them sensitive to very low levels of light. They can become 10,000 times more sensitive. Very low luminosities of only a millionth of a foot candle can be detected by some people. This is a very remarkable ability on the part of the nervous system and it is one which is easily affected by such factors as fatigue, poor nutrition, anxiety and general psychological well being, or stress.

But, the ability to detect low luminosities was only a part of what was required of night flyers. Their task was to be able to detect shapes, shadows and outlines in the dark and then to take appropriate action in regard to them. It is in the higher

centres of the brain that the messages from the eye are proc-
essed and become conscious percepts. This part of vision is
largely a matter of learning, experience, and training; and psychological factors like attention, distraction, boredom, fatigue,
and a sense of physical well being can affect visual efficiency.

Normally, in this age of artificial light, few people are called
upon to use the night vision capacity of the rod cells, unless
they should be poachers or the game keepers searching for
them. The senior ophthalmologist in the R.A.F. medical service
was Air Commodore Livingstone – later to become Air Marshal
Livingstone, Director of Medical Services – had devised a
method of testing six cadets at a time for their ability to
recognise shapes at low levels of illumination. This was done
on an apparatus known as a Hexagon. Most of the testing was
done by young W.A.A.F. officers trained as orthoptists.

My job was to run the department, to check the eyes of the
cadets and to make the returns of the results of the testing for
onward transmission to the Air Ministry. Most of the work was
of a routine nature, but there were opportunities for doing
some minor research and for finding some unusual or interesting facts relating to the tests.

These caught the eye of Air Commodore Livingstone who I
was soon to discover was a man of great drive and enthusiasm
who gave much encouragement to junior medical officers
working for him. He was a South African by birth a man of tall
stature and gifted with a ready sense of humour. He could be
intolerant of service procrastination and of ill informed criticism of his progressive ideas for helping aircrew posted to
night flying duties. So, he used to ask me to visit airfields of
various kinds to make observations for him on the spot.

This led to some interesting trips for me. One was to
Lossiemouth in Scotland where some of the earlier four-
engined bomber squadrons were being prepared to find and
bomb the German battle cruisers Scharnhost and Gneisenau in
the Norwegian fjords. The operation was one of high secrecy
and the station was virtually sealed off from the outside world
in such matters as the use of telephones or travel on leave.

At that time there were no electric runway lights, and such personnel on the station who could be spared were sent into the nearby conifer forests to gather brushwood which would be ignited at the right time to make a flare path for the take off of the Stirling and Halifax aircraft being used. It was a wild night with clouds scudding across the moon as the flames and smoke rose from the bonfires acting as runway lights. This was my first glimpse of an R.A.F. operational sortie.

Most of my assignments were to operational training units or to initial flying training stations. On a visit to one of the former I witnessed my first aeroplane crash. It was dark and a Vickers Wellington bomber was in trouble. It was being guided in with the aid of searchlights when it suddenly nose-dived into the ground and caught fire. Attempts to rescue the crew were unsuccessful as the aircraft was well alight. Nobody knew for sure whether there had been any bombs on board at the time, but small arms cartridges were exploding sending their bullets into the air. At the time I did not realise that without going through the barrel of a machine gun they had a low velocity and were not as dangerous as they sounded.

On another trip to Scotland I went to a Coastal Command training unit where they had been having some difficulties with the Blackburn Botha training aircraft. It was winter and flying was restricted by snowstorms. This meant that I could get a long weekend of leave. An old music playing friend of my mother was a laird living nearby in a typical laird's house set in an estate. I took the opportunity of staying with him and enjoying his generous Highland hospitality. He always wore a kilt and at breakfast kept to the tradition of eating his porridge standing up.

On Sunday we went to the Scottish Presbyterian Church which meant a walk over some hill tracks and alongside a loch to a village. He was dressed in his kilt with a plaid over his shoulder and a long crook-ended walking stick, while I was in R.A.F. uniform feeling very ordinary beside him. The simple service was one which I remember with pleasure. Everyone knew each other and it was an occasion for the gathering of the local clan, so to speak. Before the service the shepherds had tethered their sheepdogs in the church porch. The simple service ended with a rousing sermon from the black-surpliced minister. Afterwards there was much gossip and exchange of local news.

Then came the return walk of several miles back home to where a lunch including venison of local origin was enjoyed. Once, on going to the top of a hill behind the house, I had the thrill of seeing a golden eagle soaring up the valley below me which was a dramatic spectacle I will not forget.

At the time there was some criticism of the value of night vision capacity testing as a way of assessing its use in action, and an experiment had been designed to answer some of these questions.

A series of buoys, surmounted by different shapes or figures of a standard size, were moored in a part of the Thames Estuary near Greenwich. I was ordered to take twenty or thirty cadets to the river and to embark them on a small naval vessel the size of a drifter. After dark we were to sail down the line of buoys with the cadets recording the shapes on them as they were passed. A leading civilian statistician, Dr Bradford Hill, was to accompany us and direct the tests.

My first problem came when naval row boats arrived to take us out to the drifter. The Sergeant who I had got to come with us to keep some sort of order had gone off to relieve himself and was temporarily lost. I realised that there must be some sort of recognised drill for embarking service men of which I was ignorant. The young naval officer and his men were being very correct and smart, obviously enjoying my clumsy attempts to get the cadets into the boats in some sort of order. As things turned out conditions for the test were far from ideal: there were showers of rain and at one time an air raid further up the river accompanied, as usual, by searchlights, anti-aircraft shrapnel and sirens, but we in the R.A.F. enjoyed this unusual experience.

Once I was sent to Cranwell where some of the initial training was done. On being offered a flight over the Lincolnshire bulb fields in a Percival aircraft training wireless operators I seized the opportunity. I could sit beside the pilot and admire the view while the wireless operator behind practised his skills. I was enjoying the view when the pilot suggested that I might try my hand at flying as there were dual controls in the front cockpit. Needless to say I tended to over correct making the aeroplane porpoise a bit. That, plus some probable fear of what was happening, made the wireless operator air sick, and he opened his canopy and was duly sick over Lincoln.

Other incidents remain in my mind. There was the time when on an aerodrome in southern England a thunderstorm damaged the electrical supply to the station causing alarm signals to be sounded. The sausage balloons, trailing wires which were intended to foil any low-flying enemy aircraft, were automatically inflated and rose into the air as the alert signal was sounded. This impressed some newly arrived American Air Force personnel who were on the airfield, and we felt for a moment that we might be the target for an enemy attack on the station.

The most interesting assignment that I was given was when I was sent to a Pathfinder bomber station commanded by Air Commodore Bennett the pioneer of much of the Pathfinder techniques used by Bomber Command.

When I arrived there I had thought that my work would have been considered to be of minor importance on so busy an operational station with its high professional reputation. Therefore, I was surprised when I reported my arrival to find that I was expected and welcomed. I was told that the Commanding Officer would see me before I carried out the tests and that he would like to discuss my findings and conclusions with him before I left. The quiet efficiency of the whole station with all ranks going about their tasks with an air of purpose was impressive and made me feel honoured to have been on that station at all. It also made me eager to experience living and working on a flying field.

Besides carrying out my special duties I did my share of orderly medical officer duties, first aid training and a bit of lecturing to the cadets on health topics. The latter once led me into a difficult situation, when I was told to give a lecture on the subject of sex and its possible perils to a bunch of cadets many of whom in that intake had been policemen and probably knew much more about some aspects of it than I did. I had to stand on a stage in the Seymour Hall with the C.O. at my side and the padres from the C. of E. and the Catholic Church and Scottish Presbyterian Church on the flanks. In those days there were many taboos on too open and candid discussions on this important part of life. The wry grins on the faces of my audience as they waited expectantly to see how a somewhat raw and junior officer would cope with the situation did little to reassure me as I prayed that the stage curtains might fall on this comedy act.

Soon after Russia had joined the allies there was an influx of Polish and Czechoslovak aircrew who had been P.O.Ws. of the Russians. Many of them had suffered malnutrition and deprivation. They had been sent to an airfield near Nottingham for medical checks and assessment for flying duties. Many were thought to be vitamin deficient, and as vitamin A is essential to dark adaptation for night vision I was sent to their airfield to test their capacity for seeing in the dark. I found myself one of about half a dozen British officers among two or more thousand Polish personnel. Their own medical officer welcomed me and told me about the ordeals suffered by the Polish people. His own wife was in Paris and he managed to correspond with her by some clandestine method.

I found I had entered a vigorous and exciting atmosphere. I was told that once Hitler had been defeated the Allies should see that the Russians should be expelled from the Poland they had occupied. The eagerness of my new friends for immediate action was most impressive: but with it they retained a lively sense of humour. Their spirit became clear at an ENSA party show given by entertainers from one of their towns. Among the turns were some satires on the Allies; John Bull came onto the stage as a stout rubicund figure slow and ponderous in his movements and responses, while Uncle Sam appeared in his traditional dress wearing stars and stripes, thin in figure and indecisive, sitting on the fence. Another turn consisted of two players sitting on kitchen chairs and indulging in a lively argument in which the audience joined enthusiastically. Although I could not understand a word, I could enjoy the feeling of excitement, humour and national pride around me. For the final act there was the singing of Polish national and traditional songs in which all joined with the fervour one finds in Welsh choirs.

It was one of my most moving experiences, for here were young survivors of unspeakable horrors showing us their unconquerable spirit. This was at a time when the war was not going too well for the Allies. Since my few days among the Poles I have retained a great admiration for them and their country; they have the sort of spirit nations and individuals need for survival.

There were many more small incidents which remain in my memory. One cadet turned out to be a murderer and was eventually found guilty of this crime. He would kill young women in air raid shelters but made the mistake of bringing back with him minor trophies of his crimes which were enough to secure his conviction, and he was duly hanged. Some time later I travelled up to the Midlands on some job to do with camouflage. On the train I travelled with the detective who had been on the case, and he told me that the family had refused to make a plea of diminished responsibility despite some obvious traits of psychopathy and that the murderer had remained obdurate to the last.

One day we were visited by King George V1. Very soon he showed that his inspection was not just an occasion for smartening things up and soon to be forgotten. His probing and critical mind brought about some significant changes in the station. There was some confusion about his inspection of the medical officers. First we were to be drawn up in order of rank or length of R.A.F. service, but this looked absurd as a very short E.N.T. specialist was standing next to an enormous and tall general duties M.O. Quickly we were rearranged in order of the height which must have looked just as absurd. The King spent a great deal of time in the Mass Radiography department, which was a new form of mass screening to detect tuberculosis and other chronic lung diseases. He was impressed by what he saw and had a long discussion with Wing Commander Traill the chest specialist in charge of the screening.

Night vision testing and tests for latent squint became of increasing importance in air crew selection the former, for night flying duties and the latter for judgement of distance and height in landing aircraft.

Sometimes Air Commodore Livingstone would invite me to attend a meeting to discuss problems concerning visual performance under service conditions. After one rather protracted conference during which he did some complex doodles, he took me in to Fullers in the Victoria Road for some tea. It happened to be near closing time and he had been bored by the meeting. He was a big man with a big voice. 'Little Hay', he said, 'have you heard me do my animal and bird imitations?' 'No, sir, but I would like to do so.' With that he went through his repertoire to the surprised amazement of the other customers present in the restaurant. Many must have thought that I, an obviously junior medical officer had been deputed to care for a more senior one suffering from some sort of nervous stress. A pioneer of research into the visual problems of flying and an immensely hard worker, he had a ready sense of humour and when off duty a dislike of the pomposity common in some senior officers.

One interesting visit was to the National Physics Laboratory where work was being done to find the levels at which light just became visible. This was at a much lower level of illumination than the level at which shapes, outlines and movement of objects could be accurately detected.

Livingstone's pioneer work became recognized and accepted by senior officers in the Air Ministry including those in charge of the medical branch. Bomber Command and then Fighter Command were increasingly concerned with night operations. Then the Royal Naval Air Service became interested and I was sent down to their training and operational centre at Lee on

Solent. Arriving at the officers' mess I was invited to 'come aboard' and shown to my cabin and 'berth' though still safely on dry land. In the mess I was the only officer not in naval uniform and so the subject of some interest, and hospitality which threatened to become excessive.

One evening, I was cornered by a very senior naval officer far gone in his cups. In a very loud voice he made detailed enquiries about life in the R.A.F. and about the W.A.A.F. in particular. With his eyes becoming more tearful and glassy he boomed on about the glories of British womanhood through history starting with Boadicea and continuing via Queen Elizabeth the First up to the present. I was trapped much to the amusement of the young R.N. officers who had experienced this performance before, but not, as at this time, at the expense of a junior R.A.F. officer.

The problems to do with dark adaptation and night vision were well recognised by Bomber Command which had set up ground training centres at its operational training airfields. The effects of moonlight, clouds and shadows were demonstrated on ground apparatus, and also the recognition of different aircraft both allied and enemy types. It was found by experience that performance could be markedly improved by the use of training methods using low levels of illumination where the rod cells of the retina rather than the more central cones would be used. Speed of recognition of objects and reactions to visual stimuli could be considerably improved. I had heard rumours of these methods of training being interesting to Fighter Command.

At the same time I wanted to work on an airfield and not spend all my service life in London or in selection duties. So, tentatively, I asked Air Commodore Livingstone if I could be considered for such a posting, though personal requests for postings were not always looked upon with favour in time of war. However, thanks to the Air Commodore, I was sent to a night fighter operational training station at Cranfield in Bedfordshire as a junior medical officer with special responsibilities for the medical side of night vision training besides helping with routine station medical duties.

This posting took me into one of the most interesting and rewarding periods of my life. Sometimes I was to feel that things were too good to be true for me with so many of my contemporaries called upon to fight in deadly battles in unpleasant places. But in the services one does as one is told and with my asthmatic troubles I might have been of little use in rough conditions.

Cranfield had been an important R.A.F. station before the war. There was a spacious officers' mess with comfortable accommodation and single rooms for many of the permanent officers: there was good housing for airmen and N.C.O.s and before the war, their families in brick buildings. In wartime some of these living quarters were allotted to the W.A.A.F. and as far as I can remember only the Commanding Officer had his family with him actually on the station. Courses of flying personnel who had finished their initial training would come to Cranfield for operational training on night-fighter aircraft and the use of the latest forms of radar to guide them to enemy night-bombers.

The aircraft were Bristol Beaufighters; these were large twin-engined machines derived from the Bristol Blenheims developed just before the war. They were powerful and effective aeroplanes in the hands of competent pilots but temperamental in the hands of the less skilled. The aircrew had all been carefully selected and had scored well on testing for night vision capacity. They had a very busy schedule to follow before passing on to their operational squadrons. So, further additions to their programme like night vision training was not at first welcomed by the operational training staff or by the students themselves. Therefore it was necessary to demonstrate that night vision training was worth the time and trouble.

We had a close liaison with the physiologists of the Aviation Medicine Research Department at Farnborough, and Flt.Lt. Goldie who had a particular interest in the visual problems of flying. He was a remarkable man, a bit of the academic in uniform, but he did not hesitate to have some alarming experiments carried out on himself such as sitting in an aeroplane

with his head held in a vice while a camera photographed his
retinal arteries during such manoeuvres as looping the loop. He
would visit O.T.U.s and operational stations to lecture and to
meet the aircrew and discuss their problems with them. Sometimes he would invite me over to Farnborough to see something of his work there.

We also had one or two visits from Dr Craik of the Department of Applied Psychology at Cambridge. On one such visit
he was held at the guardroom as a suspect dressed as he was in
an ancient raincoat and tweed cap, his hair long, and clutching
a battered suitcase of papers. I had warned the guards of his
intended arrival, but when he came he did not fit their idea of a
Cambridge Professor.

Many of us can feel lost in the dark and have difficult in
interpreting shapes and shadows: optical illusions are more
apparent. It was found that Polish cadets coming from rural
farming areas performed 10% better than their British counter-
parts on the hexagon test. I was sent on visits to a variety of
airfields in England and Scotland assessing night vision problems.

Meanwhile, Bomber Command had started a night vision
training programme at its O.T.U. at Upper Heyford. The driving
force behind this was a regular R.A.F. medical officer Sqn Ldr
Kelly. His outspokenness on matters which he thought important had not endeared him to some of his superiors especially
as he was usually right as events turned out. Nevertheless, he
got full support from the Director of Medical Services, Air
Marshal Whittingham, and Air Commodore Livingstone. When I
heard that Fighter Command were to set up a night vision
training school I had asked to be considered for the post of
medical officer advising on physiological and psychological
aspects of night fighting. I did this work in addition to the
normal duties of a station medical officer. The night vision
school was set up at the night fighter O.T.U. at Cranfield. We
worked in close liaison with the Aviation Medicine Research
department at Farnborough and had the help and advice of Flt.
Lt. Goldie the medical physiologist.

Training the aircrew began with lectures, films and demonstrations. The latter were particularly important because in the course of their training they had had to listen to a lot of lectures on many subjects. The key was the Hunt Trainer which consisted of a screen illuminated from behind against which model aeroplanes were seen in silhouette. Dark adaption takes about half an hour and the aircrew wore dark goggles or red ones, as the rod cells are not sensitive to red light. They would then sit in the dark and the screen was illuminated to the levels they would find in the night sky.

At a level of 0.002 foot candles the dark-adapted rod cells take over from the cones. This is equivalent to half to a quarter moonlight. Starlight is 0.0001 ft. candles and a cloud covered dark, starless night less than this. Full moon is around 0.01 ft. c., and sunset about 35 ft. c. Modifications to the trainer included a cyclorama effect of scudding clouds to demonstrate the effect of contrast. Moonlight on the surface of white cloud could give a range of visibility of up to 7,000 feet. It was under these optimal conditions that the early pioneers of night fighters gained their successes. Finally, the lights would be switched on for a minute or two to show that dark adaption which had taken half an hour or more to acquire could be lost very quickly. We could also demonstrate the effects of dirty perspex, which could adversely affect night vision to a significant degree.

Unfortunately, both Professor Craik and Flt Lt Goldie were to die at a young age, the former in a road accident and the latter from a malignant condition. Both were brilliant men with much to give to medicine and it was a privilege to have met them.

Some years ago I gave a lecture to the local Round Table on night flying problems and night vision training. My lecture notes are appended to give some idea of our work and the reasons for it.

Station Medical Officer

Besides my special duties I was a station medical officer under a senior doctor of Squadron Leader rank. The duties consisted of taking sick parades, being a sort of Medical Officer of Health, and looking after the sick quarters which might be compared to a cottage hospital. We were also responsible for a satellite aerodrome, Twinwoods, which was some miles away and the other side of Bedford and I would go there sometimes to do relief duties.

Flying would go on both day and night and one of the doctors had to be on call for crashes, not only of aircraft from our station but any other aircraft within a certain distance of us. Therefore, we might be called to crashes or forced landings of returning night-bombers which had been damaged or of American aircraft. The high octane petrol used then usually meant that a crash resulted in an explosion or a fire which made survival almost impossible.

We had a staff of over twenty orderlies, clerks and ambulance drivers under Flight Sergeant Bateson, who was a tower of strength having served in the R.A.F. in its early days after the First World War, and then, later on in the Air Ministry as a civilian Civil Servant before being recalled as a reservist to the R.A.F. Thus he had unique experience of the workings both of the Air Ministry and the R.A.F. and he knew a lot about the characters in the top jobs. As a young man he had served in Iraq on armoured cars and while there had been with Air Commodore Livingstone. If the latter happened to be anywhere in our neighbourhood he would call in unannounced to our sick quarters to chat with Bateson about their old times together in the Middle East.

On one occasion, Livingstone was drinking strong char out of a mug and eating a thick piece of buttered toast when an irate Station Commander came in to tell me off for not having given him prior notice that this tall, resplendent senior consultant was to visit the station. Livingstone invited the C.O. to stay and hear something about the R.A.F. 'in days when you were just a boy'.

There was a large W.A.A.F. contingent with girls doing a variety of jobs including looking after the balloon barrage which was supposed to rise into the air trailing wires to entangle any low flying enemy aircraft which might raid the aerodrome. Fortunately, they never had cause to be put into action in earnest, though they were raised in practice alerts. A lot of these girls were jolly and tough women from the East End of London.

Needless to say a variety of sexual problems arose, and the Air Ministry decided to instruct the W.A.A.F. with a film on the subject of sex. A letter arrived under confidential cover to say that the film was on its way to us. At its showings no men must be present except medical staff and if no female projectionist was available the male projectionist must be out of sight of the audience. The film duly arrived under labels like 'highly confidential' and 'secret' etc:, so expectations ran high among the medical orderlies of both sexes.

The film itself turned out to be something of an anticlimax. It opened with a scene of high summer in a setting of a grassy field with a pond surrounded by reeds and yellow irises with water lilies floating on the surface of the water: the witty comments and cat-calls then started from the audience. After mounting tension, the scene changed to two frogs facing each other, their throats aquiver, until they decided that this was it and together they plunged into the water to enjoy their nuptials. It was impossible now to maintain any order as laughter shook the building and the wit of the East Enders mounted. The rest of the film was unexciting and consisted of diagrams and the expected exhortations.

In the R.A.F. museum at Hendon there is a W.A.A.F. Nissen hut which was a rest room for airfield W.A.A.F. On the outside is a notice to say no airmen are permitted to go nearer than twenty feet or so of the place, or words to like effect. The instruction I had received as a medical student on sexual problems was totally inadequate in the face of some of the problems with which I was now confronted. I knew little about homosexuality or lesbianism, though those who indulged in the latter gave us few real problems. The real difficulties came from the Americans who could give a death sentence for rape.

Once when I was on duty at the satellite station, Twinwoods, I found a girl saying that she had been raped in an American military vehicle. She was making a considerable scene and the police were there with her. I ordered her to be stripped naked before the woman police Sergeant and my W.A.A.F. medical Corporal. No bruises or injuries of any sort were found despite her vivid story of the fight she had put up in self defence.

The other case of supposed rape involving the Americans caused me more anxiety. A W.A.A.F. was reported to be missing following a dance at an American base. She was a simple girl, the daughter of a country clergyman. She was found eventually and brought back to Cranfield in a dishevelled state and distressed and hysterical. It was plain that she had had more drink than she was used to having and had passed out, after which she had attempted to leave the station by crawling under the perimeter wire. I tried to get the nearest R.A.F. consultant obstetrician and gynaecologist to help make a report on this case, but he refused to come to my aid.

Luckily, I was able to persuade the detectives on the case to drop any charge of rape and so escaped the prospect of being the only medical witness in a serious case which might have ended in a death sentence.

Flying went on at Cranfield day and night except in very bad weather or when visibility was poor. There is an element of drama on all busy aerodromes and this was particularly marked in wartime with aircraft at night taking off and landing on runways lit by flare paths. One would see them as dim shapes in the huge expanse of the airfield, and hear the screams and throbs of their engines rising and falling as they came and went on their missions. Sometimes one would be in trouble and the air control people would clear the skies on the approaches to the runway and give precedence for an emergency landing while alerting the duty fire fighters and the emergency ambulance and duty medical officer.

When forced landings or crashes occurred either on the airfield or within about ten miles of it, the alarm signals would be sounded. Sometimes we would see flames and columns of black smoke rising into the air to guide us to the scene. Then we would know that it would be unlikely that we could do much to help save the crew even if the fire-fighters were able to bring the blaze under control.

Our job then would be to search among the wreckage to find clues giving the identities of the crew members and to learn where the aircraft had come from if it was not one from Cranfield. Often the bodies would be so mutilated that it was impossible to piece together scattered bits of human flesh which we would bury under a hedge while gathering the larger pieces into sacks for subsequent burial with due rites.

When there were survivors the badly injured or burned were taken to Halton Hospital for specialist treatment. Attending at aircraft crashes was testing for the medical orderlies on whom we depended for so much. With few exceptions I was lucky, and looking at a group photograph of them by an R.A.F. ambulance recalls to me much of their personalities and the events we dealt with together.

One veteran of the First World War had been a stretcher bearer on the Western Front. Of small stature, with a marked sense of humour, he was a great stand-by in moments of stress. Despite his experience, he refused to be promoted to Corporal rank, even though I urged this on him as it meant a rise in pay. He was reluctant to take the leave due to him and on his return would ask whether there had been any crashes in his absence. I joined them for a Christmas lunch in the sick quarters and I still have the menu signed by them together with an unsolicited tribute to their feelings about our unit and myself.

All crashes were stressful events particularly when they involved aircraft from our own station, but some were due to lapses of discipline. The worst one of these shook the whole station. It involved a small, twin-engined transport plane piloted by an officer who had flown in combat in the First World War. He was a mature, cheerful person who was something of a father figure to the young aircrew in training. He was coming in to land on a fine, sunny day when he was buzzed by a Beaufighter, piloted by an instructor trying to show off to a

W.A.A.F. with him unofficially in his plane: the planes collided in the air and crashed onto the airfield causing the death of the much loved veteran pilot and all his passengers which included at least four or five American Air Force personnel.

The Beaufighter nose dived into the ground killing its pilot who was responsible for the crash and his W.A.A.F. girl friend whose body was so badly injured that it took some time to identify her. One of the Americans was still alive when pulled from the wreckage, but efforts at resuscitation were fruitless, though making the effort did something to mitigate the sense of shock the medical orderlies and myself felt; it is always easier to cope with a crisis when one is kept busy. This disaster was felt by everyone on the station, all the more so for being unnecessary.

Once, when attending at night at a crash of a large aircraft which had come down by some farm buildings, I was searching among the wreckage for human remains when I came across a tethered goat quietly munching away amid bits of burning debris as if to say 'this is nothing to do with me, and I will continue to eat as if nothing has happened'.

One incident turned out to have an element of farce about it, which was a change from the usual grim reality. We were told that a small aeroplane had belly flopped into a ploughed field and that the pilot though unhurt could not speak much English. He was dressed in a bright blue uniform and was being held by the local Home Guard as a prisoner, because it was thought that this might be another incident like the flight of Rudolph Hess to Scotland or that some sort of spy had been captured. In reality he was a Turkish air cadet seconded to the R.A.F. for training at a time when it was thought possible that Turkey might join the allies.

As time passed the demand for night vision training increased. The Fleet Air Arm became interested, and night vision schools were formed in some of their operational training stations, and women of the WRNS were sent to us at Cranfield to learn of our methods and how to use the night vision apparatus. The main aid was the Hunt Trainer, which has been described earlier.

I was able to fly at night in Beaufighters as there was room behind the pilot for me to stand and get some experience of the real problems. Although these were training flights the aircraft were armed in case of some enemy foray into England. When the plane banked, climbed and descended in sudden manoeuvres as the pilot tried to get a sighting on his radar screen I found myself suffering from considerable sensory confusion. My aural balancing sense would not integrate with my muscle position senses and my eyes would deceive me further as searchlights swept the skies. This meant that the pilot had to be able to concentrate on his instruments and make allowance for his senses misleading him to some extent.

Inevitably, the presence of W.R.N.S. on the station excited some interest and comments, especially as they were centred on the sick quarters. The opportunity came for me to visit a Fleet Air Arm training station near Berwick. I managed to get a lift in a Mosquito aircraft and enjoyed a bird's eye view of wartime England as visibility was good that day. After doing the business I had gone to do on night vision training I found myself joining in an officer's pre-wedding stag party. This annoyed me as I had become keen on one of the W.R.N.S. officers who had been sent on a course to us at Cranfield. However, I was able to enjoy some of her company the next day before returning to Cranfield. Soon after the war we were to be married.

The journey back in a naval Anson transport aeroplane had its excitements. Soon after take-off, carrying besides myself some officers going on leave with their bicycles and a dog, flares were fired from the aerodrome and we returned to land. I never knew what had gone wrong. A second aircraft was procured, and all went well until one of the engines failed and we made an emergency landing at Wittering, a large bomber station. Our aircraft had not enough power to taxi off the runway, and I was ordered by the pilot to get out and push. Needless to say, I could not budge it and the pilot was getting worried about large four-engined aircraft wanting to land after some operation.

As preparations for D Day became ever more urgent the station became busier than ever. We were sent glider pilots and low level intruder pilots for night vision training, while the engineering section was working day and night to modify Spitfires for ground support duties. From time to time I got the chance to get a flight in an aeroplane, but what I enjoyed most was being in the air in a two-seater, open light plane which gave one an exhilaration and a feeling of being at one with the elements absent for me when in a closed aircraft.

I enjoyed life at Cranfield and sometimes felt guilty about my good fortune at being there. I liked the wide open space of the airfield and the daily dramas: there were, of course, tragedies and anxieties, but often comedies, and there was constant interest in the people and work. There were professional visits to outlying units including Woburn Park where reserves of bomber aircraft were stored and guarded by aircraftmen with large guard dogs. One of the dog minders was a scion of a rich noble house with years of experience of gun dogs behind him.

Sometimes I would be in the neighbourhood of Newport Pagnell, and I got to know an old Irish horse trainer who had the traditional gift of 'the horseman's word' and who could manage the difficult horses sent for training to him. His charges would follow him around like dogs. Dressed in a horseman's tail coat and top hat, he would put on displays for charity, making his mount do paces to music and dressage exercises. One side of his house was elegantly furnished while the other side was a bit of old Ireland littered with impedimenta of horses and dogs, with a tame badger living in one corner. I had many enjoyable rides with him. Once I took him into our officers' mess at a time when we had some Australian students on the course. After some whiskies Jimmy's stories got ever more Irish and vivid, until I had to rescue him from his new found friends who were loth to let him go and asking for just one more tale.

The Station Education Officer used to invite people of distinction to give lectures. He would ask me sometimes to help him entertain them, and so I had the privilege of lunching with Sir Adrian Boult of the B.B.C. symphony orchestra, Myra Hess, the pianist, and Father D'Arcy the theologian among others. Meanwhile, the Entertainment Officer would bring to the station E.N.S.A. performers or circus artistes and entertain them in our mess.

With the allied invasion of Europe the need for more night vision training diminished and a new posting came for me.

I was sorry to leave Cranfield and the medical orderlies with whom I had shared so much of the pleasure and pain of day to day medical work. I have a group photograph of the team in front of the ambulance to remind me of so many incidents of those days.

One of my favourites among the medical orderlies was a little middle-aged man who had seen service in the First World War as a stretcher bearer. Known as Butch he was a tower of strength at the scenes of aircraft crashes, tending and succouring the survivors and ready to be close behind the fire-fighters in any rescue attempts. Although so keen on his job that I had difficulty in persuading him to take the leave due to him, he declined to take my offer of a recommendation for promotion to the rank of Corporal.

I told him to try for promotion as he would get more money to send back to his wife. He eventually agreed and appeared before the Group Senior Medical Officer to be questioned. His uniform was clean and brushed, his tunic buttons and boots shining: he gave a smashing salute to his examiner and stood to attention. Then, he realised that he had left out his false teeth, blushed, apologised, and asked to be allowed to fetch them. This comedy put everyone in a good humour and he passed with flying colours. In civilian life he was an expert cottage gardener and a standard rose I bought off him graced my mother's garden for many years.

Finally, what can one say about the aircrew themselves? All were volunteers and had been selected by rigorous test for intelligence, physical fitness, and aptitude. As individuals they covered a large part of the spectrum of human nature.

The popular cartoon figures of Pilot Officer Prune and the assertive handle-bar moustaches of Jimmy Edwards were well known parodies. In reality they were subject to great stress both in training and operations, and these stresses were too much for a few of them. Psychologically, when flying at night, particularly over enemy territory, there were the anxieties of isolation in the closed world of the cockpit. At the same time the technical demands of flying, navigation, and concentration on night flying instruments stretched the coping mechanisms of the brain to the limit. They were determined professionals, and for the most part retained a lively sense of humour and sense of proportion. They were free from the destructive emotions of rage and anger which were sometimes apparent in those nationals whose countries had been overrun.

Once when a famous night fighter squadron was threatened by a proposed visit from some psychiatrists they arranged to put on a show of bad nerves with the frenetic chewing of raw carrots*, throwing books about, or muttering inconsequential and doubtless blasphemous remarks. Unfortunately the visit was cancelled.

Perhaps a collection of Air Force poetry gives a better idea of the sensibilities of so many of them. One which has appealed to me goes as follows.

> O ringing glass
> And drowning sailor
> Some go to war
> With words on paper.
> O whistled tune
> And luckless airman
> Some go to war
> Sheathed in a sermon.
> Some are too wise
> To think it over

---

* A source of Vitamin A essential for night vision.

Or grudge to lose
Sweet life, sweet lover.
And lucky ones
Of simple nature
Kill, not to kill.
But serve the future.

That future is one that all of us have had the opportunity to enjoy.

Chapter 7

R.A.F. (Part 2)

The Posting when it came was to the Far East. This pleased me. I thought it would be a chance to see more of the world and anyway it was just a matter of time before the war was won and I had learned to control my asthma with relatively simple medicaments. I reported to a medical board in London for assessment of fitness for an overseas posting, but to my chagrin I was made out to be fit only for home or European duties. So I went to Folkingham in Lincolnshire. The aerodrome was situated on high ground just to the west of the flat lands leading down to the Wash and the sea.

It was a new station formed to serve the glider regiments to be towed by aircraft to the scenes of operations. When I arrived, there were only about a dozen officers and little more than a couple of hundred men or so. The buildings were Nissen huts and we had to set up our administration from scratch. The hut designed as the sick quarters was bare of any comforts, but a good-hearted lady-bountiful living in the area helped us with rugs, pictures, and some of the appurtenances of civilized living which we take for granted. I was told off by a Group Senior Medical Officer for making it too comfortable, and he added that the wheel castors of the beds should all be in line as if on parade. When he saw a hare I had shot in one of the rooms his face tensed and reddened until I said 'sir, I shot it especially for you'. After that I could do no wrong.

There was good rough shooting around the aerodrome and I

was able to take some of my bag up to London for my parents feeling the pinch of rationing. They had lived there through the blitz, and through the V1 and V2 attacks which were still occurring.

There was an airfield defence unit on the Wash where the men were trained with live ammunition in the firing of mortars. When called on to inspect them, I took the opportunity to try my hand at wild-fowling, sitting in wet dykes for the morning and evening flights. With me would be the Colonel seconded to the R.A.F. Regiment and a Corporal who I found had been a gamekeeper in civilian life. We would spend the night in a remote pub in the area: it was run by a large friendly lady who, a born raconteur, would regale us with eerie and exciting stories of the neighbourhood. Of course, the Corporal did best as regards the bag, but personally I was happy to enjoy the sunrise over the marshes and the drama of watching the skeins of geese, the ducks and the waders against the huge skies of the area.

Soon the station grew in the number of personnel and a medical officer with the rank of Squadron Leader was posted to be in charge of the sick quarters: this caused me a certain amount of pique as I had had all the responsibility of setting up the sick quarters and I remained a Flight Lieutenant. However, the war situation in the winter of 1944-45 was changing fast in the Allies favour, and I was due for a further move.

I was posted to the R.A.F. hospital at Rauceby in Lincolnshire for a course. There I had the opportunity of seeing something of the work of an outstanding surgeon, by the name of Braithwaite. He had made a special study of plastic surgery in the tradition of Sir Harold Gillies and Sir John Macindoe. A quiet spoken man, he worked himself unsparingly to help the airmen who had suffered severe facial disfigurement and other injuries from burns caused by high octane petrol which had been ignited in aircraft crashes, when war damaged planes attempted to land after operations.

Used as I had become to the terrible civilian injuries caused by bomb raids on Birmingham, I had to summon up my resolution in order to appear at ease with some of these patients. However, the dedication of Mr. Braithwaite, who I had seen before the war when he was a surgical registrar and I a student at St. Bartholomew's Hospital, and his trained team was an interesting and valued experience. The weeks and months of a series of plastic operations could stifle the hopes and resolution of these badly injured men.

Behind the fearful masks lacking the normal powers of expression were young human beings in early manhood with years of life before them, and now threatened with crippling disabilities and disfigurements. The damage to their self esteem, their personal hopes, and their fears of seeing family, friends, or girls, was second only to their physical injuries. The will to live and survive could so easily flicker or be extinguished by their suffering. The restoration of their morale was an important part of their recovery. Families and friends were helped to co-operate in their convalescence, and civilian visitors would come and befriend them in a non condescending way.

When the patients were better enough they were taken to country pubs after the publican and his customers had been carefully rehearsed and instructed on how they could accept these men in a natural fashion without any lulls in the talk or embarrassment at the sight of disfigurement. Mr. Braithwaite would supervise this aspect of recovery himself. He died some years ago now, but he remains one of my medical heroes.

In contrast to the realities of hospital life some of the absurdities and comedies of service life would come. For instance the padre put up a notice on the chapel which read 'abandon rank all ye who enter here', although like every padre he sported the Squadron Leader's rings on his tunic, and rank helped to make visible the responsibilities and structure of the different posts within the service.

However, over sensitivity to the precedence of rank could be tiresome sometimes. I was due for some leave at a time when a high ranking medical officer, a regular, was visiting the hospital and had at his disposal a staff car with a Corporal to chauffeur for him. Tentatively, I asked if I could be given a lift up to London with him, only to be told that it was unlikely that there would be room in the car for me. Some simple arithmetic showed this to be nonsense. Wishing to avoid the discomforts of wartime train travel I suggested that there might be room for me in the seat beside the driver. With some show of concern for me he said I could go in his car if I had no objection to sitting by the Corporal chauffeur, and this, of course, made the journey pleasanter and more relaxed for me.

My next posting was to be to Germany with the Forces of Occupation. Once again I said goodbye to old friends and arrived at an R.A.F. staging aerodrome in Kent. In a few days I learned that my destination would be to Celle in Germany. I flew to Celle in a R.A.F. transport plane, and could see something of the effects of bomb damage to the erstwhile *Luftwaffe* aerodromes. Over Germany itself many of the towns showed evidence of the effectiveness of the allies' bombing. Celle itself seemed to have escaped bomb damage, but before taking up my post on the aerodrome I spent a couple of nights at the Group headquarters to learn something about what would be expected of me as a senior Station Medical Officer of Squadron Leader rank with a junior medical officer, a Flight Lieutenant, to help run the sick quarters and deal with the day to day medical work.

Celle was a well established airfield which had served the *Luftwaffe* since before the war. Built on the sandy soil of the state of Hanover, the countryside around consisted of rather poor farmland interspersed by woodlands. Peasants ploughed the land in an old traditional way using oxen or horses, or sometimes an ox and a horse yoked together. The airfield buildings were spacious and mostly of concrete construction, and the sick quarters were luxurious by wartime standards and they included a small well-tended garden.

Refugees from Central Europe were employed on the menial tasks on the station, and I discovered that one of the sick quarters cleaners had been a high ranking Romanian aristocrat, and rumour had it that she had had the rank of princess. She had got herself engaged to a bucolic R.A. Sergeant, this being one way of achieving British nationality. There were several hundred Nazi prisoners of war, mostly *Luftwaffe* personnel, on the airfield, and they were supposed to have their own medical service, but their young doctors were poorly equipped and they seemed to have only had a brief training, and qualified more for their political attitudes than for their professional skills.

We had to take on the responsibility of supervising these men's activities. To help us with this duty we recruited a young woman who had been a medical orderly or nursing trainee during the war. She was an intelligent, pretty girl who kept firm discipline in her patients. But she could be truculent and given to ridiculing the British and to making abusive remarks. One of my medical orderlies could understand the German language, and he kept me informed of what she was saying, and this obviously had to be stopped.

At that time Germans working for the occupying forces were privileged compared to their compatriots, in that they could enjoy service rations, regular pay, and such medical attention as they might need, while outside the German civilians suffered the privations of food scarcity, disorganization of life and other uncertainties. I depended on her for my dealings with the Germans as my understanding of the language was limited.

In a sense I admired her defiant spirit when most of her colleagues were anxious to make up to the allied services to gain the shelter and benefits which the rest of their countrymen were denied in the way of food and money. So I tried to alter her attitude towards us and to trick her into a more co-operative frame of mind. I showed her some photographs of the notorious Belsen camp where Jews and dissidents were starved, tortured, and put to death. Her reaction was that these pictures were false and were composed as part of the American and British anti-Nazi propaganda. Expecting a reaction of this sort I told her to collect her things and that she would be transferred to Belsen to help clear up the mess there. I had a jeep with its engine running outside, ostensibly ready to transport her to the camp. I had no authority to do this, but my trick worked and she realised that the crime of Belsen was real. She burst into tears and begged to stay on our station. She had been in the Hitler Youth movement in her adolescence and subject to continuous propaganda.

Thereafter she became a friend to us in the sick quarters and was an excellent nurse. Once when we took a seriously ill German airman to the hospital in the nearby town, she berated the surgeon for keeping an English doctor waiting.

Later, when I had occasion to take to the hospital one of those Germans working for us who had fallen ill and needed hospital care, I had the opportunity of meeting some of an older generation of medical people, who had been trained in traditional German medicine. It was easy to talk with them and to work as colleagues in the profession without there being ideological barriers between us. They had treated British prisoners of war who needed hospital care with skill and thought.

Celle itself is a beautiful medieval town which reminded me of the scenes of fairy tales come to life. It has a Schloss with pinnacled turrets, and inside it there is a miniature theatre which was used on occasions for E.N.S.A. entertainments. If my memory is correct, we sat in small boxes amid a glittering *décor* of gilding and mirrors. Fortunately, Celle had escaped serious war damage and it has remained a place I would have liked to have revisited. There was an interesting and well kept museum which contained among its treasures some old manuscripts: in one of these was an allusion to horned hares which seemed to have mythological significance. Later I was to see a stuffed head of a hare with horns; but will say more of this later.

Nearby in the country there was a stud farm for magnificent Hanoverian horses. The stallions were fine animals standing over seventeen hands high. Despite the shortages caused by the war they had been given ample rations and were tended by devoted grooms in splendid stables. This was in marked contrast to the evidence of so much human misery and poverty in the population in the aftermath of defeat.

The human ravages of five years of war were all too apparent. Food was desperately short and roadside weeds, nettles and dandelions were being harvested by the hungry. On the railways there were long slow trains, often of cattle trucks, crammed with refugees trying to find some sort of home and shelter; many of them may have been displaced persons seeking their old homes and surroundings. There were displaced people from many countries and some of them had been prisoners of war. The currency had broken down despite the efforts made by the Allies to stabilize a German mark to avoid runaway inflation, but faith in this mark was lacking and cigarettes became a more acceptable medium of exchange. Farmers with eggs and vegetables to sell soon became the cigarette equivalent of millionaires.

Men, too, were in short supply as Germany had suffered severe casualties and many of their soldiers were languishing in Russian prisoner of war camps. Hence girls were available to our troops and would sell their favours for food and perhaps for consolation in a bleak world. As a result, venereal disease flourished with gonorrhoea and syphilis assuming virulent forms.

The country around the aerodrome was a delight with the woods rich with wild life. There were deer, and one might get an occasional glimpse of wild boar. Among the birds there were red kites and some of the black variety, while the insects included the striking Camberwell beauty besides many others rare in England.

There were ex-German-cavalry horses available for us to ride, and together with our R.A.F. Scottish Kirk padre Angus MacCaskell we would canter and sometimes gallop along the sandy tracks and roads through woods and villages. Angus was a good horseman and an ebullient character which made it quite a business for me to keep up with him, as he would give his tough-mouthed charger its head.

A lively person, Angus enjoyed expressing himself vehemently, and his theological debates attracted many to his meetings, both Christians and atheists. When a Nissen hut was consecrated as an Anglican chapel the rituals of three knocks on the door and other rites caused him to mutter fairly loudly, 'popery, sheer popery, mon'. On one occasion he had played football with such vigour that he strained a knee severely enough for me to admit him into the sick quarters.

It so happened at that time that an E.N.S.A. party from the *Folies Bergère* was in Celle to entertain the troops. Angus said he wanted to attend the show as it would be the only opportunity he would get to see that kind of entertainment which might be displeasing to the Church elders back home. So, I was inveigled to take him with me in the sick quarters Jeep. He came in full uniform including his dog collar supporting himself on crutches. I had to guide him down the aisle to where the officers sat in the front rows while he acknowledged the cheers and greetings of the other ranks with quips and repartee.

Angus was a very genuine man with a true vocation: he was a great support to anyone who wanted his advice so that we doctors never hesitated to ask him to help us in dealing with difficult medical cases. Later, although we were to live many miles away from each other, we would combine a holiday in Scotland with a visit to his manse and enjoy dinners and yarns together.

Always one for a new adventure, he told us that he had walked along a high aerial ropeway connecting two piers of the Forth bridge as he knew the engineer in charge of repairs being done on it. His wife had scolded him for being late for lunch after this adventure. She, herself had been born and bred on a Highland sheep farm, and told us that she had seen the Loch Ness monster; but she was shy about telling people this for fear of being derided. Good padres in war and in its aftermath were invaluable to us, but others could be silly or interfering in matters outside their training and experience.

There were several varieties of aircraft on the airfield, Spitfires with the ends of their wings clipped for low level operations, Tempests and Typhoons of the Tactical Air Force and transport planes of several sorts from Transport Command were landing and taking off regularly. There was an air photography unit which systematically surveyed the countryside to detect arms and explosive dumps and to gather other information of value to the occupying forces. There was a meteorological unit, and one day when I was in their station I heard a message being broadcast stating that the weather outlook was one of clear visibility and blue skies. Unfortunately, the young W.A.A.F. officer had neglected to look out of the window where a snow storm was in progress, albeit one of short duration. Littered about the periphery of the airfield were the wrecked remains of *Luftwaffe* aircraft, and I have on my desk a wooden lamp made by a R.A.F. Corporal from the propeller of one of them.

The Army Liaison Officer was Alfred Ash. His job was to follow up the information garnered by the air photographic unit and to visit the sites of interest: these could include such things as bomb and ammunition dumps, and other impedimenta of war. I formed a close friendship with him, and as he was given a generous allowance of petrol I was able to join him in some of his researches. In particular, I was able to go with him into the Harz mountains looking, not only for the debris of war, but also seeing an area rich in historical and literary allusions.

Bad Harzburg was made into a resort for troops on short leave, and it was possible to enjoy there various sports including horse riding and, in winter, skiing. In fact, a German prisoner of war who had served in the Nazi alpine troops and was also a trained parachutist, had been put in charge of the skiing activities acting in the role of a professional ski coach. I found that in the course of the war he had been to places in Norway which I had known and where I had had some pre-war skiing holidays. We enjoyed chatting together about the places both of us had known. This was another example of the futility of war for so many individuals who, devoid of feelings of personal animosity, are caught up in the machinations of politics, dogmas, and the abstractions generated by narrow minded institutions.

But, Alfred liked to get away from the military milieu, and with his enquiring mind and the wiry physique of a long distance runner, we made some strenuous expeditions in the Harz mountains. He had to investigate an area high in the hills close to the Russian zone of occupation which included the highest peak in the range, the Brocken, which comes into Goethe's Faust.

Alfred had become friendly with an old German inn keeper called Herr Kuhne whose family had suffered badly in the war, especially towards the end when there had been severe fighting in the woods around his home involving crack Nazi storm-troopers in a sort of last ditch stand. He was of typical peasant stock with a balding round head and bushy moustache. He was welcoming and grateful for our gifts of tobacco and food. He told us that he had been a game keeper and forest ranger. Certainly he had a good knowledge of the animal and bird life of the Harz.

In the hall, among mounted heads of deer and boar, was the head of a hare with small horns rather like those of a small roe deer; I took some photographs of him holding the horned hare's head, and one of them was published in *The Field*. Though I am sure that this was a fake it stimulated some controversy among naturalists for a time. But, the question might be asked as to why go to the trouble of faking a horned hare. The Harz mountains are rich in folklore, and hares figure in mystical and pagan religious traditions in several countries including Ireland. As has been mentioned earlier, there are references to horned hares in ancient manuscripts in the library in Celle.

Alfred discovered from Herr Kuhne that one of the oldest mines in Europe was nearby, and with his interest in geology he decided that we should visit it. Guided by an elderly, lame miner holding a lamp lit by candles we entered the labyrinth of passages to be shown the mineral strata. It would have been all too easy for our guide to have extinguished the candles leaving Alfred and myself to be lost without trace in the depths of the mountain. Fortunately, Alfred and our guide, lost in the details of the mine's history, were too busy to bother about such things as the recent war and the state of European politics.

On another occasion when exploring the Harz from Herr Kuhne's inn we found a village with a mining museum. It had been shut during the war, but a proper approach to the caretaker and the discreet offer of cigarettes persuaded her to open it up for us. It was a beautifully displayed life-size reconstruction of early mining practices and the ways of the miners. Despite the war, it had been cared for lovingly and every detail was in place. First we were shown the chapel where the miners would pray before descending to the work faces by a rickety system of ladders. In the porch, coats and hats of the seventeenth and eighteenth centuries were hanging on pegs, and inside were hung by the pulpit the numbers of the hymns and psalms to be sung in the service. The pews and primed oil lamps looked as if they were still in daily use.

After this we were taken to the mine adit and saw the twin ladders which, moving up and down alternately, would hasten the descent to the working face and the subsequent ascent at the end of the shift. Underground, were life-size models of men at work, and at one place there was a reconstruction of a mine disaster with a roof fall crushing miners caught under the debris. The attention to detail was impressive, and this was the first historically reconstructed exhibition of active life in the past which I had seen, though nowadays many museums show dramatically how life might have been lived in earlier times.

Goslar is a delightful little medieval fortified town and had an officers' club graced by a genius of a chef who applied his skills to the stodgy, if substantial, service rations. He had been captured by Montgomery's men and pressed in to the job of looking after officers on short leave, a post he seemed to appreciate where he could practice his culinary skills and enjoy our appreciation of them.

Among many in the services there was a certain sense of anti-climax with the war having ended, demobilization under way, and men's attention being directed towards the problems of the future in civilian life, though at the time life was pleasant and easy in Celle. In the spring the storks flew in to build their nests on the cartwheels which had been placed by people on some chimney pots. From the windows on the top floor of the R.A.F. hospital where was the medical officers' mess, we could watch the activities going on in the stork nursery, from the building of the nest with piles of sticks, to the hatching of the young and their growth and development.

Some people and incidents of those days remain in my mind. At one time I had become friendly with a middle aged R.A.F. officer who was stationed at Group Headquarters. He was a bachelor, an erstwhile city business man, and a member of some of the best London clubs: he was also an epicure. When the menu was right he would invite me to dine in the officers' mess at Group Headquarters. The dining room was large and had a minstrels' gallery where a small, German music group would play mostly classical music to us. It also boasted an excellent wine cellar inherited from some of the top brass of the *Luftwaffe*.

Once, when at the next table to us were some senior R.A.F. officers my friends suggested that we should send up a note to the musicians asking them to play the Twilight of the Gods. This they did with relish, though Wagner's music was supposed to be forbidden to Germans. There was some consternation as to whether or not this piece was by Wagner and whether it should be stopped. Some thought that Wagner epitomised the soul of Germany and that his works should be suppressed. My friend was a brave man as his job was to investigate and arrange for the disposal of numerous German arms dumps, and these could include anti-personnel bombs like the so-called butterfly bombs easily detonated by slight tremors or movement. Despite this he seemed to enjoy his work which required a rare and calculated form of cool courage.

Celle was the place where some of the German guards of the notorious Belsen concentration camp were taken for standing trial for war crimes. In the surrounding countryside there were some armed bands raiding farms and outlying houses for loot. Many of the members of these gangs were ex-prisoners of war captured by the Germans from a variety of countries and who had been turned into forced labour slaves. They were rounded

up eventually and brought to justice. One night in the officers'
club in Celle I found myself hob-nobbing with a senior Polish
officer who was a prison commandant; he was also very drunk
and I could not easily get away from him. Embracing me like
an old and intimate friend he told me how he had either shot or
hanged six men that day and was now celebrating the event.

Germany was a crushed and destitute country with cities
such as Hanover being a mass of rubble and ruins from intensive bombing. Public services had broken down and they had
to be taken over and run by the services of the Allies. This
applied to medicine to some degree, though those hospitals
still functioning did some very good work with the medical
staff and nurses working long hours at a time with limited
facilities.

However, the situation was often different in the country
areas, and in some cases the Germans had nobody to call on in
emergencies. This meant that we had to help out and go to the
rescue of German civilians when it was a matter of urgency.

So it was that one evening there was a case of obstetrical
difficulty in a nearby hamlet. Luckily, an R.A.F. ambulance
plane had landed on the airfield that day with a nurse on
board, and I was able to enlist her aid. Off we set in a jeep with
my Flight Sergeant and a medical Corporal. We found the girl
in an exhausting and prolonged labour lying in the middle of
an enormous continental bed which I had to climb onto in
order to assess the situation.

Our German language skills were not up to the demands of
the problem and various members of the girl's family were
being busy and fussing in unhelpful ways. Efforts to get some
sterile boiled water eventually resulted in an old lady carrying a
bucket of water who started to scrub the floor with vigour.
Then all the lights went out, the power station being in the
Russian zone of occupation. The jeep with my highly excited
Flight Sergeant went back to our sick quarters to fetch more
torches.

Eventually the baby was safely delivered among emotional
scenes from the girl's family which included an elderly, nerv-

ous and silly old man who dithered about giving out orders to his women folk. As I looked up from the bed I saw on the wall a framed picture of a stern faced Nazi officer in full uniform with an icy glaring expression to match. I suddenly realized that this family hero was none other than the now deflated and interfering old man. Before we departed I turned the picture face to wall as a mild gesture to show that we did not want any more reminders of Hitler's dream fantasies. Mother and baby were transferred in a R.A.F. ambulance to a German hospital and both did well.

However, I was to have more trouble from this incident. My Flight Sergeant of the time was a rather silly man too big for his boots. He gave a highly dramatic and inaccurate account of these events to a lady journalist dressed in R.A.F. uniform whose brief it was from a London evening paper to get 'human stories' about the doings of our troops in Germany. I had the greatest difficulty in stopping her from forwarding a tendentious article which would have been embarrassing for us: I had to muster up what threats I could think of from the doctor patient tradition of confidence to holding her responsible in a disciplinary sense for any inaccuracies coming from her pen.

In June 1945 I was due for some home leave, and I had arranged to get married during it, although my future was uncertain after being over four years in the R.A.F. and the uncertain future for the medical profession as a health service would be introduced within about a couple of years. What sort of service it would be depended on whether a socialist or a conservative party was in power at the time. Anyway, I was fairly far down the list for demobilization.

Just before I went on leave I had given some medical attention to a Finnish girl who had been in the German equivalent of the W.A.A.F. She had been given a job of waitress in the officers' mess: I had asked her how it had come about that she had found herself a P.O.W. with the R.A.F. It appeared that her father was a prominent man of affairs in Finland, and her family had escaped to the Germans in preference to surrendering to the Russians who were invading their country. When the

Allies had arrived at the airfield she had taken refuge in a cellar as she had been told of the savagery of the British and Americans.

Once she had realised that we were not as cruel and vengeful as she had been told she settled down as a popular and attractive member of the mess staff. But she had lost contact with her family and knew nothing of their fate. I put her in touch with a Quaker organization which was trying to help refugees. When I returned from my leave she came up to me in an exuberant mood with my dinner plate filled generously with the best of the day's menu. She had found her parents and was in communication with them. As everyone knew I had just been married, her greeting to me was the cause of some leg pulling.

I did not see much of my home or parents on this leave as most of it was spent honeymooning by Exmoor, horse riding and enjoying life free from the nagging anxieties of war. By now I was desperately keen to have a home we could call our own. I had spent years living as an institution inmate in school, college, hospital, and the R.A.F. I had had some wonderful experiences and met many fine people, though this had been balanced by the anxieties and uncertainties of war. I had learned, the hard way, a great deal about people for which my education had not prepared me.

I felt it was time now that I should live my own life within a family. I had reason to suppose that I could have stayed on in the R.A.F. from hints dropped to me by P.C. Livingstone, now an Air Marshal. But I was still prone to asthma and had still to use drugs to control it and had to dissimulate about my health problems.

Soon after my return from leave I was given another posting in Germany, this time to Fassberg, an airfield situated in remote heathland with patches of forest dotted about. It was a Tactical Air Force station commanded by one of the R.A.F. ace pilots. The squadron flew low level attack Tempests and Typhoons in ear shattering and nerve wracking evolutions. It was also a station where the *Luftwaffe* had been experimenting with a variety of rocket propelled planes, and there was a test bed for firing tests horizontally against an inclined concrete mound to try out different fuels.

At the time there was some competition between the Russians and the Americans and the British to get control of German research establishments. Captured German scientists were offered contracts and advantages to themselves and their families if they continued to work for their captors. Werhner von Braun, who later helped to develop the American rocket industry, was in charge of the research at Fassberg. He, and others, had been allotted pleasant houses with many privileges denied to most of the Germans. I visited some of them in their houses and was received with a courtesy rare in England with their sons bowing as we shook hands, and their daughters giving little curtsies.

To investigate the scientific work and to supervise the research some distinguished British scientists were dressed up in uniform and posted to Fassberg. Among them were some young ladies in W.A.A.F. officers uniform who were really technical assistants to the senior men.

At the time there were one or two squadrons of the Belgian Air Force on the station. The men had managed to escape from the Continent during the war and they were robust, daring and energetic people, though often harbouring feelings of hatred towards Germany that was of an intensity unusual in the R.A.F. At a mess party one evening they began to sing their special songs which got wilder and more drunken as the evening progressed. At one point they took off a garment at every verse. Before the climax arrived some of the more prudish British officers tried to hustle the ladies out of the mess to the annoyance of some of them. Nowadays in like circumstances the ladies would probably have been offended at not being able to witness the bare truth as the final chorus rang out.

Sometimes potentially dangerous experiments or low level flying demonstrations were to be carried out and the medical section would be ordered to attend with ambulances and emergency equipment at the ready.

One of these occasions was when there was to be an attempt to increase the range of V2 rockets by cooling their engines with liquid oxygen. We medicos watched the proceedings from a slit in a concrete wall many feet thick. The suspense grew as a bowser of liquid oxygen was wheeled in on rails and the rocket engine primed. Previously I had only seen liquid oxygen poured in small quantities from a thermos bottle by chemistry demonstrators at my university. The tension rose as the rocket engine failed to fire and I felt some relief when told that the test would have to be postponed, as I doubted whether the concrete would have proved thick enough if everything had gone up in an explosion. Later the experiment went according to plan.

The Tempest and Typhoon squadrons which specialized in low level attacks and the so-called skip bombing wanted to show their prowess to senior army and air force officers, and a demonstration was arranged using live ammunition. The targets were captured German tanks and lorries filled with captured German explosives to give dramatic effect. The top brass were to witness the show from a grassy mound at what was supposed to be a safe distance. The first pilot armed with a rocket banked steeply for his run in, but unfortunately he pressed the button as he was banking and the rocket flew low over the heads of the spectators, and one had the experience of seeing a variety of senior officers lying prone with their hands upon their heads. The rest of the demonstration was noisy and dramatic, and it gave one an inkling of a few of the horrors to come in later wars.

I became friendly with one of the British scientists and went with him on several trips including one to see my old friend Herr Kuhne. This scientist, whose name escapes me, was a senior adviser on chemical matters to the government. I found that he was what I would call 'a fellow traveller' in the communist tradition, and although friendly and courteous on a personal level, his political theories included some very callous mass suppression of those who could not easily accept the Leninist line. I had before regarded intellectual political theorists as being of little importance from what I had seen of them at my university and medical school: now my mind was changed and it remains changed.

In the sick quarters I found that I had inherited a fine Alsatian dog; my predecessors acquired it from Belsen concentration camp when that was demolished. It had been a guard dog. It was a splendid, intelligent animal and I enjoyed many walks with it, but it had been trained to make nasty noises to civilians in mufti, though it was reliable with anyone in uniform. When my turn for demobilization came I left it with the airfield defence police.

There were still some armed bandits around, and once driving back in the dark from Celle to Fassberg, I found my jeep confronted by men with rifles waving a torch at me. I felt very much alone on that road surrounded by heathland. I changed into low gear and with the headlights on drove at them on a zig-zag course hoping to frighten and confuse them. As they jumped out of the way I was hailed by an English soldier who, having lost his way, had managed to join up with an allied patrol who said they would wave down any passing vehicle to help him.

Near the sick quarters a stream ran along one of the airfield boundaries, and I found that it contained a good stock of trout. On some evenings I would manage to catch some of them, and handed them over to the orderlies. Much to my disgust they turned them into traditional fish and chips dishes.

The shortage of food made it important that as good harvests as possible should be gathered, but the farmers near woodland suffered from the predations of wild deer and boar. We were asked to organise shoots to cull the game. R.A.F. airmen were not skilled rifle men, but armed with military Lee Enfield rifles, the sportsmen would stand near the edge of a wood as beaters with much noise drove the quarry towards the guns. This proved to be a dangerous sport as the hunters themselves were at risk from stray shots from the enthusiastic sportsmen.

Once I went on a dusk deer shoot, and sat uncomfortably in a tree. As evening came on the deer emerged from cover and one started to scratch itself on the trunk of the tree I was sitting in: I preferred to watch it rather than to shoot it at close range. However one of the party bagged a deer: being medical it was thought appropriate that I should disembowel it, a task I performed with distaste and inefficiency. Then we had to fit the carcass across the bonnet of the jeep and drive back with a dreadful stench being wafted back in our faces. This cured me of any hunting instincts I might have possessed, though for a few years I would enjoy rough shooting of birds for the pot before I sold my father's valuable shot-gun without any subsequent regrets.

Chapter 8

Back to Civilian Life

Leaving the R.A.F. after nearly five years service meant one of those big changes in life which come to most of us from time to time when our directions, purposes and meanings assume new shapes, and the road into the future is an unknown quantity. I had been lucky in the R.A.F. with my postings, my work and my colleagues, but I had come to realise that I was becoming a sort of institutional-inmate-person who could never say 'this is my home, my furniture, my life'; one was always at the disposal of a higher authority. Moreover, the spectre of asthma could not be suppressed for ever with the limitations on physical activity and confidence which it imposed.

I had spent years in boarding schools, university, hospitals, and the forces, so the dreams of being a private person were attractive, as such dreams should be. Besides, I was now married to complete the dream. Before the war I had taken it for granted that a physical disability would make me unacceptable to the kind of girls whose company I enjoyed. I had never been completely at ease on social occasions or skilled in the social graces.

My outlook remained middle class professional, and the pressures to conform to what was considered to be a good career were strong. I was getting older and time was running out on me if I was to have any chance of finding a satisfactory niche as a civilian doctor with younger, newly qualified men and women graduating from the medical schools and whose service commitments were comparatively brief in duration.

So, I declined to follow up a strong hint I had been given that I might apply for a permanent R.A.F. commission. The R.A.F. was changing: old friends were leaving on demobilization; wives and families were beginning to come out to Germany and the life of a peacetime garrison was taking shape with many of the old wartime challenges gone to be replaced by duller and more routine ones.

Another officer and myself were detailed to be in charge of about two hundred men on their way home for demobilization and a return to civilian life. Needless to say there was a general air of euphoria with less respect for discipline, so that herding our flock to Hamburg and then aboard a Liberty ship for an overnight voyage to Hull was no picnic. From Hull they were to go on a special train to Leeds. On the way the train broke down and several men got out onto the tracks to be left behind when we got under way again. We were relieved at saying good-bye to them and to resume our journey to the officers demobilization centre at Cannock.

There we were well treated and handed out good quality civilian clothes. We were ushered into booths according to our physical shapes: I was told to go into the one labelled 'tall and average', while a much more senior officer was expostulating angrily at being ushered into the 'short and portly' one. The issue of ration cards brought us down to earth as we realised that we were no longer privileged service men in regard to food and clothing.

I had arranged to take my wife to Switzerland as a kind of second-half of the honeymoon we had enjoyed a few weeks beforehand. In 1939, as I have said, I had left Bergun just before war broke out and the Swiss were mobilizing to defend their frontiers. As I had said farewell to the proprietor and his family and staff and we had wished each other the good fortune to survive the impending catastrophe, I had sworn that I would return to their hotel in happier days. This was a dream which never faded in the intervening years and I had determined to keep this promise to myself. The weather was beautiful, the Alps majestic and serene, and the people generous in their welcome to us. The food had all the savour which Swiss culinary expertise had made famous: and all this after years of war seemed a miracle as if the good things of the past could continue and get even better.

Days of walking in the mountains finding the wild flowers and stalking chamois, and marmots to watch them about their business, and even seeing the ibex of the Engadine all made impressions as lasting and beautiful as any in our tablets of memory.

In our last week at Bergun we had arranged to climb one of the local peaks with the aid of a guide. The weather nearly let us down as we made our way to the hut at the edge of the glacier we were to traverse next morning. Walking up the track through forest we found ourselves in increasing darkness and mist until we emerged suddenly onto an alpine meadow with a clear moonlight sky above us and the snow-covered peaks standing out sharply around us, while below the valleys and forests were invisible under a magnificent white cloudscape.

After a few hours of sleep we set off over the glacier to the foot of the Piz Ketsh which we were to climb. Our guide was a large, elderly man of the mountains like someone out of a storybook. He had lived and worked all his life in the area and was one of those people kindly, efficient and good humoured who enjoyed introducing tyros like ourselves to the mountains he loved. We were roped together before crossing the glacier as there is a danger of falling into a hidden crevasse; in fact a boy from our hotel had done just that and died. The final rock climb was steep but not difficult. The wonderful panoramic view over the Engadine which we had from the summit was all the more magnificent in its grandeur after the fears and horrors of the war years.

To be, just us three, in such surroundings gave me once again for the moment something of that 'oceanic' feeling of ultimate confidence and reassurance, which reduces so much of human concerns to their true proportions. Maybe, this is all a delusion, but it is a delusion worth having and is the opposite of futility.

The aftermath of war had left England poor and exhausted: food and clothes were rationed, while nearly every big industrial city had been scarred and had buildings destroyed by the bombing raids. There was much jostling among demobilized service personnel to gain a footing in civilian life which might give them the prospect of a successful future: often there was a tinge of envy towards those who, through poor health or a reserved occupation, had not been conscripted and were already well up in their work or professional ladders. As is so often the case the doctors had been in a privileged position; they had been doing medicine in the services and Aneurin Bevan's Health Service was about to be born and would need all the medical power available to run it, however hard the difficulties of adjusting from the old system might prove to be. Times of transition are times of anxiety mitigated by new opportunities: but it would be necessary for us to adjust ourselves from the traditional outlook in which we had been trained to a new system of state-organized medicine.

Service doctors had lost touch with civilian medicine and in particular, the care of children and the aged, and of obstetrics. The purchase of an established practice from a doctor who was retiring would be expensive especially as the buying and selling of practices would be abolished once the new Health Service became law.

I was fortunate in obtaining an ex-service training post at the Birmingham Childrens Hospital which had became famous for its work under the guidance of Sir Leonard Parsons the professor of paediatrics. Essentially, I was once again a student attending clinical ward rounds, out patient sessions, and lectures. After some years of carrying my own responsibilities I found this to be a bit of an anti-climax, though I was catching up on a branch of medicine in which I had become rusty. The winter of 1947 was very cold, and we were living in uncomfortable rented rooms. Food and transport were limited and we had no car as cars were in short supply and there was a waiting list for them even if one could claim that one's work gave one some priority. Birmingham seemed to be a rather depressing place with its areas of bomb damage and buildings dilapidated from lack of maintenance and repairs.

At the hospital I became friendly with a Palestinian student who introduced himself saying 'I am George Attallah, that is what you would translate as Theodore, the Gift of God'. I could only reply that my name was Michael Hay and that the surname meant dried grass. Unrealised by me this exchange of names was overheard by Professor Smellie who had succeeded Sir Leonard Parsons.

George was staying in digs and was feeling upset because his landlady had, for some reason, refused to cook the rice he had brought to England with him and which he had acquired from the region of Syria; he had heard that we were short of food here and he had wished to supplement his rations. We offered to help him by inviting him round to supper with us which was to include some of his rice. George was, and remains, a large ebullient person with a great store of energy and a sense of humour. This started our friendship which continues after forty-four years with regular exchanges of letters and meetings when his travels bring him to England.

When at last spring came and the snows had melted, we took George to a point-to-point race meeting near Warwick. The sun was shining, the grass green and growing, the sky was blue with white fleecy clouds adding contrast and variety. The lively, well groomed horses, the good natured, keen spectators enjoying themselves, and the excitement around the bookies' stands all thrilled him. After some confusion putting on bets with the bookies, as George thought we should haggle in the eastern tradition, we went to the Tote. George was lucky and he made some good winnings.

Afterwards we went to tea with an old friend of mine in one of the Elizabethan houses close to Warwick Castle. We all had had a good day and felt the efforts for survival which had been made in the grey, war years were bringing in happier times. But, I reminded George that there were less pleasant aspects of life in leafy England, and I arranged for us to visit a coal mine.

I could do this as I had become an assistant to Dr Dorothy Campbell who was in charge of the Research Department of the Birmingham Eye Hospital. Part of her work was investigating the causes of miner's nystagmus which could cause problems of eye fixation and giddiness. We travelled to the mine on the top of a bus as I had no car at that time. George had just returned from a trip to Paris where he had met an uncle of his on a business trip. For entertainment they had gone to the *Folies Bergère* which had impressed them enormously. A loud and vivid description of the night's events enthralled the other passengers on the bus causing one or two to fail to get off at the stop where they had intended.

In the mine we tramped along the underground passages for what seemed to be miles eventually to reach the coal-face. By then I was feeling guilty at having led George into an uncomfortable experience with all the dirt and narrow tunnels. But, when we had arrived at the coal-face where coal was being loaded onto a conveyer belt, George seized a shovel and joined in while announcing 'I think I must be the first Arab from Jerusalem to hew coal in a British mine'.

The miners were delighted and later we joined some of them for lunch in their canteen. This day, too, had been a success. George became the leading paediatrician in Jordan: he did a lot of work for the Palestinian refugees and he has travelled to many countries gathering information on child health and attending international conferences on the subject.

But, 1948 was a time full of uncertainties in regard to the future, and the medical profession was still awaiting the introduction of the National Health Service with some degree of apprehension as to what changes that would bring to doctoring. I was still trying to adjust my professional life from service medicine to civilian practice. So I arranged to return to hospital work as a junior resident medical officer to bring myself up to date and regain some confidence. I got a suitable post at Dudley Road Hospital in Birmingham on another ex-service scheme. Before I went there I had time to spare, and I went on a course on obstetrics at the famous Rotunda Maternity Hospital in Dublin.

This was my first visit to the Republic of Ireland, and I was soon to become fascinated by the atmosphere of a country which had not been directly involved in the war which had recently ended. However, they still had food rationing though this did not seem to be strict as regards farm produce: the girl in the ration office was welcoming and chatty. Having found out from me that I was going to the Rotunda, she said that I would be wanting to take home some butter and eggs and told me where I could get them.

Around the centre of Dublin there were some horrifying slums, but the people seemed cheerful despite their living conditions. A bus driver on one of my excursions recognised me and greeted me: he had been a mechanic in the R.A.F. and I had evidently treated him for some complaint. He asked me round to meet his family and I enjoyed a convivial evening with him in their home. The country around Dublin was beautiful in the spring and summer and I enjoyed several expeditions exploring it.

Once, when I was on a train returning to Dublin from a visit to an archaeological site, I got chatting to a farmer who, thinking no doubt that I was a rather ham tourist, started to regale me with all sorts of legends and tales of 'Old Ireland' mixed with stories of the 'little people' and other occult beings. Not wanting him to get away with this I replied with some old English and Scottish stories until we were lost in exciting fantasies of a past world. The time passed in a cheery atmosphere, and when the train pulled up in Dublin we shook hands warmly expressing hopes that we would meet again to exchange more good stories.

One of the students on the course was an earnest American doctor, who kept himself busy by making written notes of all that came to his attention in Ireland. He came to me once because he had been puzzled by the sight of young army conscripts in the streets and had asked a passer-by what they were doing and why they were there. He was told that they were the brutal British soldiery keeping down the poor oppressed Irish – the Irish Free State had been established years before then. He could not see that he was a victim of the Irish sense of humour and love of a good story.

As qualified doctors we were sometimes asked to go out with unqualified students on domiciliary visits. This could mean visits to women in labour living in what seemed to me to be appalling conditions of poverty and general dereliction: some had evidence of undernourishment. Nevertheless, they would seem cheerful and were good patients as they brought yet one more child into the world blessed by the Catholic Church.

The teaching in the world-renowned Rotunda Hospital was thorough and practical, and I enjoyed my stay there.

There was still a month to go before I was to start work at Dudley Road Hospital in Birmingham. So, I went to a practice in Hereford as a locum tenens. It was the summer of 1948, just before the coming of the National Health Service, and I thought that I would gain some useful experience of general practice in a cathedral city with established traditions not yet over-whelmed by the industrial revolution.

The practice served panel patients who were insured through their work and also private patients. We did our own dispens-ing in a small dispensary in which I found, to my consternation, that the scales for weighing drugs were inaccurate. Most medi-cines were made up in liquid form and put into standard bottles scored with measures in teaspoons. After being corked and instructions written on sticky labels put on them, they were carefully wrapped in white paper and sealed with a blob of sealing wax at the top; later they were called for by the patient or delivered on a home visit. All this was time consuming and fiddly compared to the quick writing of prescriptions which is the way of things today.

Hereford seemed to me to be a mixture of people living in distinct spheres of life: some looked towards the cathedral and its precincts for their hopes and certainties in life: the growing professional and business communities were beginning to be more concerned with the complex profit-motivated world we know today. At the bottom of the heap were those living in as bad slum conditions as I have seen anywhere.

Once, on a wealthy estate by the river Wye, I visited the home of a farm hand looking after a family of children on his own as his wife had died. They were living in a derelict barn without any supply of running water or proper sanitation. Help for him and his children was difficult to procure despite the fact that his employers were wealthy landowners with salmon fishing rights on the Wye. They seemed not to care about their employees' domestic difficulties and plight.

On market days gypsies would turn up at the surgery. They were honest and straight with us as they fished out seven and sixpence from voluminous petticoats before they said what they wanted to see us about. We visited patients in their homes in the countryside within a range of up to ten miles from Hereford. Motoring along the highways and byways in summer was pleasant and our destinations might include anything from noble houses to dilapidated cottages. This was time consuming and sometimes I would have to return to a remote area which I had just visited that day. Nowadays radio telephones have obviated some of the frustrations caused by late calls.

The old cathedral town ways of life still persisted in some odd ways. The doyen of the senior practitioners used to go on his rounds conveyed by horse and trap. He, and his equally elderly coachman were always turned out immaculately as was the whole equipage, the horse, trap, and harness gleaming while the doctor and groom wore bowler hats and their legs were covered with a traditional horse rug. A whip was carried at the correct angle.

If I had been a patient I would have felt honoured indeed to have been visited by a doctor arriving in so distinguished and elegant a way. I felt shamed by the ropey old car put at my disposal for visits, though it was recognised as the practice car by policemen and others with a salute or wave.

One of the patients I used to visit regularly remains one of those I do not forget. Normally, in those days, babies born with severe brain defects had no chance of survival as far as adolescence, but I found myself faced by a teen-aged lad huddled up in bed, incontinent and making inarticulate and moaning sounds when approached. He was paralysed in all four limbs, and could not feed himself.

Despite all this his mother had devoted her life to him, washing, feeding, and turning him over in the bed at regular intervals without any regard to herself: her husband had left her, but she was cheerful in her self-appointed task and appeared to be free from resentments. She was unwilling for her boy to be admitted to an institution or to have professional nursing aid in the form of the district nurse. At least she had found a purpose in life which would have been too much for most of us to bear.

Midwifery was a bit of a worry to me as I had had only a comparatively brief experience of the subject, although I had assisted or been present at some difficult labours. In Hereford most babies were born in their parents' houses, or sometimes, among the wealthier classes, in private nursing homes. If I was in some doubt about the progress of a labour I could get some assistance from one of the local G.P.s who had special experience of obstetrics. This would mean usually that he applied forceps while I administered chloroform from a drop bottle in the old fashioned way.

But problems could arise which were not allowed for in textbooks or in hospital training. I was called to see a woman in the third stage of labour who was losing blood from a retained placenta. It was midnight and she lived in a remote country cottage. It seemed plain to me that she needed hospital care and I sent for an ambulance after giving some first aid treatment. On the way back the ambulance broke down in a lane without a building in sight. I had been following the ambulance in a car, and once more had to do what I could while the ambulance driver tried to get his engine going again, delving under the bonnet in a driving rainstorm. Eventually, to my relief we got going again, and our patient, once in hospital, did well.

The next worry, in an obstetric case was when I was called by the proprietor of one of the big hotels to say that premature illegitimate twins had been born in a bathroom. The parents of the young mother wanted the problem dealt with privately, quickly, and not in the local hospital, as their main concern was to avoid scandal. After ringing round to various nursing homes to be told that they were either full up or that they did not accept that type of case, I did manage to persuade the matron of one of them to admit the mother and her twins.

In those days there were no intensive care units for babies born prematurely, but the twins were wrapped in cotton wool and kept at the right temperature in a cot near a gas fire in the matron's sitting room. She fed them at frequent intervals using a fountain pen filler until they were able to suck. When I left Hereford they were doing well and the matron had become fond of them. The mother and her family showed no interest in the twins who were marked down for a children's home when fit to be moved. I would have loved to have known what became of them later in life, and they must be well in to middle age by now.

Like all communities Hereford had its saints and sinners. Among the former there were nuns living in a closed community and we were medically responsible for them in any illness. It was with some trepidation that I entered the convent on my first visit to them. But my fears were soon allayed as the sisters were charming and helpful: I could not have wished for better patients.

There were also the sinners varying from amusing rogues to dangerous characters. Among the latter there was a dark, taciturn ex-service man who drove a taxi. He complained of severe headaches which, he said, were sending him round the bend, stopping him from sleeping and upsetting his temper. I could not find any physical cause for his symptoms, but I let him ramble on. Such medicaments as aspirin did nothing to help him, but I thought he should be kept under review.

One day he came into the surgery and told me his story. He was involved in the dilemma of an eternal triangle love affair and felt that he had been grievously wronged. Brooding in his taxi at the railway station while waiting for important trains to arrive, he had determined to solve the problem with the aid of a German Luger pistol he had acquired in the war. His tenseness and look of grim determination alarmed me, and I began to wonder if I might not become a victim if I did not mind my Ps and Qs with him. After a while he quietened down as I tried to show sympathy and concern while pondering on what to do if violence was to be avoided.

Eventually, I persuaded him to throw the pistol into the river Wye and come back to me when he had done so. Much to my relief he agreed to do this, thereby resolving his problem of thoughts of revenge on his rival. A few days later he returned to say that his headaches were much better and he brought me a chicken and some eggs as a present, and it was a generous one in those days of rationing.

Sometime after I had left, a young doctor in the practice was murdered by a deranged patient in the waiting room or surgery; so perhaps it was as well that I had not applied for the post of assistant with view in that practice. Anyway, I did not think that I wanted to spend the rest of my working life in Hereford although I had enjoyed my time there. The long-distance motoring in winter on visits and having to live up to being a bit of a public figure in the busy community did not appeal to me. Also, I did not want to commit myself before I had some idea of what the N.H.S. was likely to entail.

So, in the late summer of 1948 I went to Dudley Road Hospital in Birmingham as a resident medical officer under Dr George Hearn. I still had to postpone the day when I would have a house and home of my own, but houses, money and opportunities were still in short supply. My mother, now a widow, needed some help in settling her future and winding up my father's affairs.

It was harder on my wife who stayed with friends in Birmingham, while I went back to an active life in a busy hospital as a junior trying to bring myself up to date. Several of us were ex-servicemen in the same boat and we have remained friends through the years which have followed.

Dudley Road Hospital like Selly Oak Hospital had started life as a municipal hospital and was growing rapidly into the busy, modern teaching hospital it is now. Its history has been written by Dr George Hearn who kindly signed my copy of the book. Some of the fascinating facts in the book are the stories of how much is due to several outstanding personalities in both the medical and nursing services. Their clear vision of urgent needs, together with a patient and persistent sense of purpose to meet them, brought about rapid changes to the great benefit of the community among which were many living in under-privileged conditions.

The hospital dealt with a great variety of medical, surgical and obstetric conditions in a great variety of patients, including immigrants of different racial and cultural origins who had arrived recently from what had been parts of the British Empire. The work was demanding, but most interesting: besides taking in emergency cases of all sorts, and the usual run of more chronic patients needing investigation, our unit cared for the patients of a chest surgeon who had set up a surgical thoracic unit.

Open chest surgery was a relatively new development in surgical technique needing expert anaesthesia. Nowadays heart and lung operations have become common and routine in specialized surgical units, but the experience of witnessing these operations and helping in the post operative care was new to me.

The demands on the hospital were increasing rapidly, and new developments in medical science were bringing with them new knowledge and new treatments which had to be mastered. This increase in workload was not matched at the time by an increase in the medical staff, so sometimes after a busy day we were called on to do emergency anaesthetic work late at night or in the early hours of the morning. Some of these emergency cases were extremely sick people who really required the services of an experienced consultant anaesthetist and not those of junior residents: I remember that once I ended up giving almost pure oxygen to a man already unconscious with a perforated peptic ulcer. This state of inadequate staffing ended with the coming of the National Health Service.

I had hoped to get enough experience at Dudley Road to enable me to attempt to get a higher medical degree, the M.R.C.P. But, I was unable to do sufficient book work for this, and I was still worried about finding a permanent niche in the medical world.

The birth pangs of the N.H.S. were considerable and Lord Moran the president of the Royal College of Physicians and erstwhile medical adviser to Winston Churchill took it upon himself to proclaim that on the ladder of medical worth and achievement general practitioners were on the bottom rungs. I resented this greatly as my father had been a general practitioner and I had learned something of the scope of that work. I went for interview to several practices, and was attracted to one in a remote area in the Norfolk countryside, but I thought that village life might pall as the years rolled by and that we might miss intellectual stimulus and recreation.

As so often happens when one feels down on one's luck an unexpected opportunity came my way when I got an introduction to Dr Dorothy Campbell who was a consultant ophthalmologist and the director of research at the Birmingham Eye Hospital. She was interested in my wartime work in the R.A.F. on night vision problems and she was looking for an assistant in her newly established research and biochemistry department. I had done some ophthalmology at the Corbett Hospital as a house surgeon among my other medical duties and the idea of getting myself involved in research projects appealed to me. At the time the laboratory was poorly equipped and there was some urgency in getting work started.

Migraine is a common disorder and sufferers from it would often go to an eye hospital as they could have alarming visual disturbances for which adequate explanations were lacking. Dr Campbell had an interest in the subject and I thought, though I was mistaken in this, that it might be a road into research into allergy which had plagued me for so long.

As a student, I had once asked a medical lecturer why people subject to migraine would sometimes pass more urine than normal with an attack. I had been asked not to ask silly questions, even though I knew this could happen from what a relation, subject to the disorder, had told me. In those days the label 'a functional condition' was stuck onto many conditions which could not be explained rationally. Dr Campbell agreed that this could be a relatively simple matter to investigate without the need for very expensive apparatus. I had seen references to instability of fluid balances in migraine and in asthma in a book published in 1873, *On Megrim, Sick Headache and some Allied Disorders* by E. Liveing. Miss Eva Tonks was the biochemist with a lot of experience in her profession.

There were other reasons why I puzzled over this relatively common affliction. Quite obviously anyone with a history of classical migraine was turned down for flying duties by the R.A.F. But there were borderline cases where men keen to fly had suppressed a history of episodic headaches.

One of these was an experienced test pilot I had got to know quite well and I had played squash with him. One day in summer when the sun was shining in a blue sky I was called to an aeroplane crash. I found a wrecked Spitfire aircraft with bits of it scattered over a wide area. The pilot's body was unrecognisable and mangled, but I recognised my friend by a pipe with a carved bowl which I knew belonged to him. There was no reason why he should have gone out of control at about 10,000 feet and hurtled into the ground. He had not reported anything to be amiss to flying control and he had not attempted to use his parachute.

Now, I suspect that he might have had a severe migraine attack in the cockpit. More recently a friend of mine got killed on an M road by hitting the barrier, turning the car over and coming off the road: no other car was involved and the sun was shining on a clear May day. Now, many years later we have more evidence as to what might be behind such accidents in the form of sensitivity to glare and flicker to which migraine sufferers are prone.

My wife and I were able to rent a pleasant, top floor flat in a house belonging to some relations of hers. It was a quiet area, but was easily accessible to the city centre. I would spend the days at the Birmingham Eye Hospital seeing something of the work Dr Campbell was doing on a form of blindness or defective vision known as retinitis pigmentosa. She was working also on the problem of coal miner's nystagmus which is a distressing condition causing problems of visual fixation and balance. This led me to see something of the mining industry. I liked the miners I met and admired their fortitude which their work required. The traditions of their trade and its dangers demanded a strong community spirit.

On some evenings I would go back to Selly Oak Hospital to go on ward rounds with Dr Adolf Nussey the senior consulting physician whom I had got to know when I was a resident in the hospital in 1940. He is one of the finest all round physicians I have known with an acute brain and a perspicacious sense of humour. I also did some relief surgeries in general practice.

Cars were still in short supply and the waiting lists long unless one could claim priority on account of work necessity. However, at week-ends we would explore the countryside travelling by public transport as far as the hills of the Welsh borders; in particular we enjoyed many weekends with Mrs Lloyd at Stourport, and I would go rough shooting in the woods around overlooking the Severn river as her family owned some of the land above the west bank. When, at last I was allotted an Austin ten saloon car, it became easier to visit my mother now living at Bishop's Stortford in Hertfordshire.

In the summer of 1949 we decided to drive up to Loch Maree in the west of Scotland for a holiday. My time as an assistant to Dr Campbell was ending, I had acquired some varied experience of civilian medicine since leaving the R.A.F. and the N.H.S. was getting over its birth trauma though still in a very immature state: so I had decided to seek an entry into general practice and at long last begin to live a more settled life. I found a vacancy advertised as an assistant with view post in a Birmingham suburb. We could live above the surgery and I could continue my work for an M.D. degree by completing my thesis, and could continue to see migraine patients at the Eye Hospital on a sessional basis.

Chapter 9

General Practitioner

In 1949 my long term prospects were still uncertain, and the N.H.S. had been established for about a year. I got an assistantship with view in a practice in a southern suburb of Birmingham. We were still living in the same flat in a house owned by my wife's relations, and this was four or more miles from the practice which meant longish drives at night to deal with any night emergencies.

My partner-to-be lived above the surgery which was in a three storey Edwardian brick building and which had been the local doctor's house for many years. It even had a speaking tube at the front door connected to one in the bedroom so that people in trouble could talk to the doctor in his bed. There was a large garage at the end of the garden where a horse and carriage had been housed before the advent of the motor car. I was assistant to a doctor who had bought the goodwill of the practice before the war and who had run it with assistants while he served in the R.A.F. The out-going assistant was a lady doctor who had carried a great burden in the war years and who had now decided to take Holy Orders as a nun.

The owner of the practice, whom I will call J.K. for short, was keen to move to a house outside the city boundaries and to try to form a new practice in what he considered to be a better class area. When he moved out I could take over the flat above the surgery. This was large and spacious and as I paid a reasonable rent it was useful not to have to find capital to purchase property.

Having no brothers I still felt some responsibilities to my widowed mother and to my sisters who showed no desire for marriage. There were some other advantages which I could have if I were to settle into the practice: I could continue to do sessions at the Eye Hospital on migraine, and I could enjoy the advantages of having many good professional friends and contacts in a city with two universities and a lively intellectual life. Moreover it was simple to leave the practice area and to become a private citizen on one's times off. The leafy Warwickshire countryside was in easy reach, and not too far away was the Severn valley, and westward from that the Shropshire hills and the Welsh Borders. Soon we would become members of Olton Mere sailing club which gave us recreation in pleasant surroundings.

I continued to work on my thesis on migraine and submitted this to the Cambridge University medical faculty. Much of the writing, typing and revising was done between the hours of six and eight in the morning before breakfast followed by the morning surgery and practice work.

Eventually I went up to Cambridge to be examined on it and to do a ward round with the professor: all were dressed in appropriate academical garb. The examination was conducted in a courteous way rather in the mode of a professional consultation than in the less elegant mode of my qualifying finals. At the end Professor Whitby told me that I had passed and asked me when the time came for me to be presented for my degree by him, who would lead me up to the Vice-Chancellor, not to treat his finger like a piece of cold fish, as several of us were to be led up together each clasping one of his fingers.

The ceremony was in February 1951, and at last I could feel really entitled to call myself 'doctor'. My mother came up for the presentation of degrees in the Senate House, and I have a photograph of her dressed in a fur coat outside that building. I felt that this was some reward to her after all the care she had given me in my boyhood and the worries and disappointments she had suffered on my behalf. My old college, Gonville and Caius, entertained its new doctors at the High Table, and I was able to enjoy the good food, the good wine, and good talk which is part of the life of the Senior Common Room. It was tempting to ask myself if I could not go into research and get a D.Ph. in order to get this experience again.

By now I was a general practitioner in the young N.H.S. which was still cutting its teeth and was the subject of much clamour among politicians, the press and the profession. The war years had left people exhausted by the efforts needed to defeat Hitler, and many had anxieties about their futures with problems over careers and housing. Whatever service life had meant to men and women, nobody had been on their own, and each would have filled an allotted niche and known what was expected of them. There had been close comradeship and the satisfaction of feeling wanted and playing a part, even if a minor one, in a great historic drama.

So much had been expected of civilian life, and the concept of the Welfare State promising fuller and healthier lives was very much in people's minds. The Beveridge plan of health insurance for all was popular, though the planners had miscalculated its cost which was to rise rapidly as medical progress with the development of new and expensive technology grew apace.

General practice was to continue on a contractor basis and was at a lower status than that of hospital consultants. Such things as X-rays and common pathology tests could not be requested without reference to a consultant. It seemed that medicine in the N.H.S. would operate in a hierarchical structure. It looked as though Lord Moran's ladder of achievement with general practice on the bottom rung was here to stay with the blessing of the bureaucracy of the Ministry of Health. Needless to say the rungs of the ladder were rewarded financially according to their level. Many doctors felt bitter and frustrated as was shown by their letters and articles in the British Medical Journal of the time.

In 1949 there was no general practitioner trainee scheme, and on entering general practice as an assistant with view to partnership one was expected to do more than an equal share of the work, especially as regards out of hours emergency calls. The medical schools had been consultant orientated and there had been no adequate training for general practice. In a manner of speaking I was thrown in at the deep end. On duty during my first Christmas in the practice I was called to deal with a baby, one of twins, found dead in its mother's bed, which meant an inquest and suggestions that the baby had been deliberately smothered.

In the evening I had to see a doctor living nearby with a stomach complaint. An ardent Catholic, he had constructed an elaborate crib scene on a table with national health cotton wool to give an impression of winter snow, though the figurines were in arabic dress with sandals. In the centre of the piece there stood an empty whisky bottle like a monstrous factory chimney rising from a pastoral surround. The doctor was drunk, and had to be got to bed, though with difficulty, amid protests, and offers of Christmas cheer, and arguments.

Promises made in the war about what the Welfare State would do for people formerly deprived of adequate health care had given rise to high expectations which had been damped by the continuation of food rationing, a housing shortage, and uncertainties about employment and careers. The country was impoverished and depended on American Lend-Lease arrangements. So the ailments caused or exacerbated by stress were prevalent, and doctors were expected to work miracles of healing: their failures could cause resentments and disappointment.

The pattern of diseases was different to what it is now. We saw cases of rheumatic fever in the young, and there was quite a lot of tuberculosis around. As more people were signing on to the National Health Service the numbers of patients on our list increased and it was necessary to employ an assistant doctor. The first of these was a pleasant lady doctor who lived with her husband in the flat above ours. They left after about six months or so and another married lady doctor with her husband, a teacher, came in their place.

Unfortunately he was a sick man and no doubt suffering from what we would now term post traumatic stress syndrome from his war service, though as things turned out there was also an organic problem. His symptoms took the form of anxiety states and neuroticism which he tried to counter with drugs and alcohol. The drugs were in the form of bromides which were readily available and were advertised on buses and hoardings as Relax-a-tabs. It was easy to spot the bromide addiction as he would come out in an acne rash. One day he was brought to the surgery drunk or drugged with a bottle sticking out of his pocket at mid morning. The police who were guiding him announced that he had given his name as Dr. Hay, and they had to be disillusioned by me.

I had liked the chap when I first saw him, and as he was a teacher at a famous public school, I had naively thought that I might be able to have the odd game of squash or a swim at the school in the holidays. I had to ask for a consultant psychiatric opinion, and he was put off work: meanwhile the headmaster was trying to sack him and wrote to me asking me to back him up. Knowing something of my patient's war record and that some of the boys at the school had tried to tease him, I wrote a somewhat sarcastic letter to the headmaster of the school criticizing its moral atmosphere and indiscipline while making it plain that in any dispute I would take my patient's part. We succeeded in preventing any dismissal though the time came when it was advisable to get my patient to give notice himself.

Quarrels soon broke out between husband and wife, and on one occasion a grapefruit missed its target and crashed through the window facing the street causing all sorts of speculations among the patients as to what was happening. In time there was a divorce and our assistant's health broke down. Unfortunately, an eminent consulting psychiatrist to whom I had referred my patient had not done an electro-encephalogram, which might have given the clue to the presence of cysts in the brain from which he died in another town.

Professional partnerships are not always happy affairs and mine was no exception to this. The senior partner was spending more and more time in the better off Warwickshire end of the practice leaving most of the busy end of it to me with the assistant who at the time had not been given the prospect of a partnership, although the practice was growing: also there remained a considerable difference in his and my income. I was tempted to set up on my own, but partnership agreements forbade practise within a three mile radius if the practice were dissolved. However, some irregularity in the accounts gave me the chance to bring our differences to a head and a new agreement was drafted giving me the right to continue on my own in the same area, or to continue in the old practice as an equal partner and to live in a private house away from the surgery.

I did not relish being in a single handed practice and I did not want to face too many difficulties in starting afresh, so I agreed to the second course. Any future assistant was to be given the prospect of a partnership. It was to be some while before a suitable partner was found.

The first assistant with view was a pleasant lady doctor who was married to a doctor who was one of the most bigoted men I have met. He found sin in the most unlikely places including a book of medical history with early descriptions of diseases which I had inherited from my father. He seized this and destroyed it when he found his wife reading it. On Sundays he might call for her at daybreak to drive to somewhere far to the north to hear him preach. With one thing and another, she fell ill and was nursed by my wife.

The next assistant was a man who had been a missionary in China. He turned out to have some tiresome obsessions particularly in regard to dirt: this caused a washing mania and even door handles had to be wiped with an antiseptic cloth after being handled by patients and others. He, too, became ill: this time with cancer. This was successfully treated, but on recovery he went into public health.

The penultimate assistant with view came to us with high credentials from a nearby hospital, and he had a house in the area. He found the vicissitudes of general practice a strain, and he developed a psychosis of alternating mania and depression. The latter state was relatively easy for us to cope with, though it meant more work for me; but the manic phases were much more difficult.

One morning there was a knock on my door and a very angry, puce-faced, middle aged midwife complained that he had got into her car parked outside and made improper suggestions to her, and she asked me what I would do about it. He also made some fanciful boasts to patients on his doings in high society. I had to face him with his shortcomings and say he must either have psychiatric advice or leave: fortunately for us he left. Soon afterwards we heard he had died from a heart condition exacerbated by his chain smoking.

The practice was in an essentially suburban area of a major industrial city. The patients came from a wide spectrum of society but the majority were in family units and owned their modest houses. Many of the men were skilled artisans, conscientious and responsible people, but five to ten per cent were chronic cases of various kinds who gave us a disproportionate amount of our problems, which could be social as well as medical ones. They covered a wide range of diseases and disorders which could bring severe domestic difficulties to the families as well as to the patients themselves; but as the years went by we could watch how families grew and developed which is a privilege of general practice. Even in retirement I still hear from some at Christmas including, in one case, the latest family photographs.

A sense of humour is important in general practice as it can enable one to stand back and view a tiresome situation in terms of a television comedy. My old R.A.F. padre Richard Amphlett prayed for a sense of reality, a sense of proportion, and a sense of humour. These have often been a help in some tricky situations.

Many instances come to mind like Miss M. a large, florid patient subject to epilepsy who would console herself by singing loudly in the waiting room until a knock on my door would bring in an anxious patient to warn me that something was amiss: and I would suggest that others should join in the chorus and be cheered as well.

There were, too, the tragedies which one was called on to share with the families. A fine recording of the Verdi Requiem was given to me by the husband of a talented young artist who had a fatal cancer. My memory is enriched by many events and personalities with whom I have been concerned, and in retirement I value them.

Among the older patients were men who had seen action in the First World War. One of these was Frank. He needed a good deal of medical attention for a bad heart among some other ills. He was living on supplementary benefit and found it difficult to provide for his wife and children. He was always cheerful and in the course of his occupational therapy provided me with woven wastepaper baskets and a woollen bedspread done in a sort of crochet work. He had fought on the Somme and had been a stretcher bearer until wounded by shrapnel in the pelvis. He had made a good recovery and after the war he went to India and joined the Viceroy's mounted guard, being present at many great Imperial occasions. He had never made any claim for his war wounds, and I thought he should have a pension for them.

There was some suggestion that not all the shrapnel had been removed: so I arranged for an X-ray which showed bits of the shrapnel still present. With the aid of an orthopaedic consultant and the British Legion we managed to get him a better war pension, but soon after this came in, his supplementary benefit was reduced. I helped him to write an angry letter to Mr. Harold Wilson, then the premier, but this only got the usual bland reply. When his last hours came his mind reverted to the Somme and he was calling for more stretcher bearers before dying peacefully some hours after the nightmare had passed. I had enjoyed visiting him in his house and hearing some of his vivid reminiscences.

Then there was old Mr. George S., a cheerful man in his eighties with a bad chest. He had chauffeured generals around the Western Front in the First World War and had kept a photographic record of his adventures. I would look at the sepia pictures in his albums showing bewhiskered generals seated in open Vauxhall and other cars: at the end was a picture of him celebrating the Armistice in Boulogne with his arms round a French girl who was wearing his army hat. I wish we had a record of some of his stories and chat.

To listen to some of these old people in their own homes was to enter into the realms of social history and to appreciate the rapid changes in life which have taken place in comparatively few years.

Emergency calls at night were always a trial, and when on duty I would go to bed alerted for a telephone ring which might mean an emergency. In the early hours of the morning one's brain is not at its best, and one could feel very lonely dealing with a difficult problem surrounded by anxious relatives. In the early days drugs and equipment were not as refined and available as they are today.

On one occasion I was sent for in the early hours of the morning to see a man who was thought to be in the throes of a heart attack. His pulse was weak and irregular and his breathing poor to the point where he needed artificial respiration. At the time I thought that this was more of a gesture than anything else. After a while he showed evidence of recovery and his breathing became regular. A neighbour who had been a nurse sat by him while I went home for some breakfast.

When I returned I found him conscious and talking. The room was full of relations and friends who belonged to an evangelical sect of religion. There was much chatter which was disconcerting when I wanted to keep a clear head: and anyway I dislike acting in medical dramas before an audience. So I asked my patient what he remembered of the night. He said that he had been in the presence of the devil and he thought that he had more to do to expiate his sins. That could only have meant me as the devil. After this we cleared the room of his friends and we got him admitted to hospital where he made a good recovery.

Often we would give up to seventy items of service a day, though many of them were simple like repeat prescriptions, but each meant some degree of care and responsibility. The great majority of patients are co-operative and understanding, but a small number are not so and they can be demanding and unreliable taking up an undue amount of a doctor's time and attention. Some of the most difficult were the drug addicts and the chronic alcoholics, particularly when they deny having a problem and have no great wish to change their habits.

Once I was asked to see the uncle of a patient living a prosperous family life in a pleasant suburb. What I could not understand was a long palaver about 'Uncle' who had not registered under the N.H.S. I was shown photos of him in cricket gear as a member of a high class team, and I was told all about his business interests and directorships. I was given the address, and when I arrived in the road I thought that I had got it wrong, because the house with the number I had been told was dilapidated with filthy windows. I rang the bell and the door was opened by a dishevelled oldish woman, grubby and unkempt, with wrinkled sagging stockings and worn carpet slippers: the house stank.

I was asked abruptly 'what do you want here?' After some lengthy explanations I made my way to a back room keeping my overcoat tightly around myself and avoiding brushing against dusty articles of furniture. I found my patient lying in a bed on the ground floor by a window overlooking a large garden gone wild. At my heels a terrier dog was yapping. Then, as I approached the bed salvation came from an unexpected quarter. In a large cage with filthy sawdust on its floor there was a large macaw: 'what will you 'ave; what will you 'ave', it shrieked. Alcoholism was the obvious diagnosis, easily confirmed by examination and appropriate tests. Then came the business of mobilizing the public health authorities and the social services to try to save this unfortunate couple from further trouble and degradation.

These awkward patients were always a challenge and they gave me some valuable insights into some aspects of human nature; and in retrospect there was often a humorous side to these demanding crises and difficult people: in my mind's eye I could see again some of these people and events in terms of T.V. dramas.

Looking back over the years there were many tragic cases which will never be forgotten, and I remember heroism and cheerfulness in daunting circumstances. One young woman with two young sons, who was at a terminal stage of a cancer, elected to return home from hospital to die in her own home and under our care. Her uncomplaining courage and her cheerfulness made visits to her a privilege which I still value after many years.

On a happier note, there were cases of unexpected recovery from severe illness. In particular there was a little girl aged ten years with an abdominal tumour thought at the time to be incurable. It was inoperable, though a small sample – a biopsy – was taken to confirm the diagnosis. She was sent home to die in the care of her family and friends.

After a time she got bored and wanted to go to school. The headmistress was helpful and understanding, so it was arranged for her to go part time. She improved and the tumour appeared to shrink, until she could live a normal life for a child of her age. When she was eighteen, she asked for some routine tetanus vaccine as she was about to start work as a dental nurse. She let me look at her tummy and there was no trace of a tumour.

I reported this to the hospital where they had her records, but got no answer. This annoyed me and I sent the details of the case to a cancer registry, and got a most interesting reply together with a request for two eminent consultants to travel from London to see the girl. Fortunately she was a cheerful person and I explained that her case had things to teach doctors which might be of value to others. She laughed at this and said that she had never expected to be so important and was happy at this suggestion.

Years later, when I had retired from general practice, she took the trouble to look me up. Now she was middle aged, with a family and a daughter training to be a nurse. She was enjoying a busy life including running a small-holding as a hobby. This happy case history had kept me wondering and some years before her unexpected call on us I had organized a meeting on the subject of 'unexpected recovery' in the local faculty of the College of General Practitioners.

Some of my colleagues in other practices had cases of various kinds which had done better than could have been hoped for according to accepted medical teaching. We invited some pathologists to join us and had some lively discussions. We should always note those patients who survive against the odds as they have much to teach us.

Soon after the lady I have mentioned came to visit us I wrote a short essay entitled 'Survival against the Odds', and this was published in a medical journal. I included in it some of the experiences of ex-service men who had undergone horrific times in Japanese prisoner of war camps or on the long march from Poland as German prisoners when the Russian armies were advancing. These survivors have a quality of spirit at times of adversity which can teach us all a lot of valuable lessons.

The early years of the N.H.S. were not happy ones for general practice, but certain far-sighted doctors got together to form a College of General Practitioners. They sought to raise academic standards and to encourage research. Meetings, symposia, and discussions of wide ranging topics were initiated. I joined our local faculty quite early on and met some outstanding colleagues. Eventually I was honoured by being asked to be chairman of the faculty board and later provost. When in office I tried to arrange meetings which got us outside the lecture room and the hospital. One of the most lively was one on 'Farm Medicine' when rural practitioners, vets, farmers and pesticide manufacturers met together on a farm and could see farm workers in action between the discussions and papers. On another occasion we gathered at a large factory, as in a sense all G.P's. must have some concern with industrial practices. Then there was the time we had a meeting with the police and the fire brigade who put on a realistic mock show of the heavy rescue teams in action. We invited casualty surgeons to join us. When we met at a nearby spa famous for its treatments of rheumatism and arthritis we all ended up in the brine baths, which got us cheerfully relaxed before an excellent dinner.

Eventually the College got Royal Patronage and now has a high standing in the medical schools which have departments of general practice alongside the other special departments.

Looking back I feel I have been lucky to have lived through exciting times of change and to have played a small part in these events. In terms of meaning, purpose and value, I feel that the patients have given me as much or more than I could give them. Again, thanks to modern inhalation therapy, asthma was more of a minor inconvenience to me than anything else, though I had to hide it and dissimulate by retreats into the lavatory or other shelter if it should become obtrusive.

It may appear to be trite to comment on the rate of change in society as the years pass and in medicine constant adjustments have needed to be made to meet new popular assumptions and habits. Nowhere had this been more difficult than in the field of sex. In my young days it was almost a taboo subject in our middle class society, and it was closely associated with ideas of sin if one did not keep to the rails.

Divorce was talked about in hushed whispers and I was told that divorced persons were not accepted at Court.

When the chaplain, who was also the singing master at my preparatory school, suddenly went off to South Africa and some of his favourite pupils left, the reason remained a mystery to us, and quite certainly we were given no warnings about abuse of children.

As a medical student clerking in the venereal disease department made me open my eyes to some aspects of life of which I was woefully ignorant. Later as a qualified doctor in the R.A.F. the sexual problems became more intrusive. There were angry letters from parents of service women who had become pregnant and who we had sent into special hospitals for unmarried mothers to have their babies. There must have been homosexual problems, but fortunately they were not brought to the attention of the medical service. I knew of lesbian relationships in the W.A.A.F., but they caused us little trouble and where necessary they were dealt with by the W.A.A.F. officers.

Since the last war there have been enormous changes in sexual habits due to the contraceptive pill and some feminist movements seeking for abortion on demand. In my student days the procuring of abortion was a criminal offence except for health reasons. Later it was necessary for two doctors to recommend this treatment in each case, and the criteria for it were broadened. Being myself old fashioned by modern standards I would demur at co-operating on request, and I know of several children now grown up who owe their lives to my obstinacy. A doctor friend of mine was defeated in the final of his village tennis tournament by a lad whose life he had saved from being aborted. This gave him joy in defeat.

Attending cases of abortion induced by back street, unqualified practitioners could be harrowing. On one occasion I was summoned to a house where the daughter was thought to be a case of abdominal emergency. In fact she was in the throes of an abortion. Her parents and friends were gathered in the next room armed with flowers and fruit for the patient and rightly concerned about her. They belonged to a strict religious sect and I was faced by a probing inquisition before I could manage to get the patient off to hospital and dispose decently of the products of abortion.

Human children take many years to mature, and they need prolonged care and help in adjusting to life if they are to fulfil themselves in later years and become adult emotionally as well as physically. So the sexual revolutions from about the sixties onwards have brought new problems in the psychological spheres as well as in the physical ones to the medical profession, and now there is AIDS to cope with.

The immigration of people of ethnic origins other than the Caucasian also brought some new problems for general practitioners, though speaking personally I enjoyed meeting them and experiencing new outlooks and ideas. Some had stories to tell of long journeys and hardships endured before they could settle in this country.

There have also been changes in patterns of disease. Rheumatic fever is uncommon now, and antibiotics have made osteomyelitis and mastoid infections rare: tuberculosis is nothing like as common as it used to be. Once when called on to give an after dinner speech I pointed out that the Chinese ideogram for 'crisis' was a blend of 'danger and opportunity'. At that time there was the usual anxiety about changes in the N.H.S., but there must be constant change and development to avoid mental stagnation and to have the ability to meet new challenges. Anxiety about projected changes is understandable when one is already busy, but there are opportunities to be seized as did the founders of the Royal College of Practitioners at a time when medical morale was low.

Migraine

After I had entered general practice I continued to maintain my interest in migraine and was able to do sessional work on the subject at the Birmingham Eye Hospital. Although I had thought that one of the main factors causing attacks might be allergy, I soon came to realise how complicated a subject migraine would prove to be.

Some time in the 1950s I got in touch with Peter Wilson who, himself a migraine sufferer, had founded the British Migraine Association. Peter was a solicitor who had served in the Royal Navy in the war. A determined and energetic man with a fine sense of humour he would follow any likely or unlikely clue with vigour. He asked me to be a medical adviser to his association, and I agreed to help him provided my name was not put on his association's notepaper, as another doctor's name was on it and I did not want to get involved in controversy with him as I shunned this sort of publicity.

There came a time when Peter wrote to me to say that his association had collected some funds and that he would like suggestions as to how they might be spent. At that stage I felt that we needed the help and experience of different branches of medicine and the views of eminent consultants and research workers. I had got to know Dr. Robert Smith who was doing work for the Wellcome Foundation and who had done research with Professor C.A. Keele on pain. He agreed to organize a symposium.

The symposium was held at the Wellcome Building in London on 8th July 1962.

The meeting was chaired by Professor Linford Rees, a distinguished consultant psychiatrist. He emphasised in his opening address the complexities of migraine. He had discussed this with two professional colleagues on the day before the symposium and said 'It was most interesting and valuable to me to hear their personal experiences, which revealed a multiplicity of factors which can operate in migraine and also the very interesting variety of phenomena which can be observed'. The opening paper entitled 'The Consumers End' was given by Lady Snow (Pamela Hansford Johnson – the novelist). She spoke eloquently of the misery and humiliation felt by sufferers from this complaint, and her words are reproduced below.

'Sufferers will try to conceal and deny an attack because of its effect upon others. When one has been suffering from migraine for a long time, and has observed the effect upon husband and children and friends one knows that one is going to be a nuisance to them, however sympathetic they may be. A maddening thing is that whenever you have something important to do, or whenever there is something to which you are particularly looking forward, migraine may most likely rob you of the capacity to carry out your task or to get pleasure out of the treat.

'The result of this is that your family, when you are waiting together to go to the function so eagerly anticipated, cannot fail to remark the terrible strain upon your face. The strain which says – "I have migraine coming, but I shan't admit it". They know what is happening as plainly as if you told them outright. So the sufferer goes on pretending that he has not got this revolting thing, until finally he has to give in and lie down. In my case, it is often impossible to conceal the pain, because one eye is streaming tears.'

I said that from my experience the factors which seemed to contribute to the onset of attacks were fatigue, menstruation, allergy, excessive sensory stimulation, functional hypoglycaemia (low blood sugar), infections and debilitating illness, food sensitivities, and various other factors including weather and climate changes.

The meeting was a success and the speakers agreed to keep in touch with each other by means of small, informal, evening gatherings at the Wellcome buildings. Then Robert Smith got the interest of Lord Brain the eminent neurologist. Under him a Migraine Trust was formed to promote scientific research at institutions which had the means and technical facilities for the kind of research required. He became the first chairman of the Migraine Trust which has since grown and through its symposia has gained an international reputation. I was honoured by being asked to be a member of the medical advisory committee, which would meet several times a year in London.

Lord Brain was the leading neurologist of his time and he was also a philosopher and literary man of distinction. It was a privilege to have met him and this led me to read some of his essays. One of these is entitled 'The Need for a Philosophy of Medicine': in it he writes 'the characteristic feature of our present epoch in medicine is the growing significance of the idea of transaction. Many of the most important things that happen in the body can no longer be explained simply as the result of the interaction of two or more organs, but require the conception of a dynamic transaction which itself integrates the activities of the organs'. An analogy would be the poor functioning of a car engine, which could be due either to a mechanical structural fault or to it being out of tune.

Research on migraine was showing increasing evidence of the body being out of tune as regards physiological functions at times of attacks. In my student days we had been taught medicine by eminent consultants who emphasized the concept of disease with physical signs and pathological changes which were fixed relatively as compared to the rapid changes in migraine with integration being restored by sleep and rest.

Among the factors which appeared to precipitate attacks of migraine were tension and fatigue. During my time in the R.A.F. I had seen many instances of anxiety and fatigue causing mental and physical medical problems especially in aircrew coming to the end of a dangerous tour of operational duty. Often the symptoms would become manifest when the tour has ended. I had also learned that fatigue due to the expenditure of energy at a party could cause a measurable deterioration of night visual capacity on the following morning. In the 1950s H. Selye and others were doing research on the effects of stress on the body, and it seemed to me that it might be an important factor in precipitating migraine attacks.

I was fortunate in getting an introduction to Mrs. Jane Madders who was a lecturer in health education and a qualified physiotherapist. From her student days she had been interested in methods of relaxation. She introduced me to the work of Edmund Jacobson on the relation of anxiety to muscular tension which people could be taught to control voluntarily. She had done work for the National Childbirth Trust with pregnant women, and with children, and with Olympic swimmers among others. She agreed to help our migraine clinic with group relaxation classes.

These were popular with the patients largely because of Jane's personality and beautiful voice. There would be a discussion in the session and patients could find it easier to unburden their minds of anxieties in the relaxed atmosphere she would create. I mentioned her work at the first Migraine Trust symposium and showed some slides of her methods. Later we gave a joint talk at another of the Migraine Trust symposia, but it took some years before relaxation therapy became accepted more widely by the medical profession which tended to rely on tablets for treatment and to ignore other aspects of migraine.

Jane was kind enough to ask me to write a preface to her book *Stress and Relaxation* and this has been reprinted and translated into other languages.

This happy collaboration and friendship came to a close late in 1990 when she died of a heart attack. Characteristically, Jane had asked for a party of her friends and co-workers as a commemorative memorial. This was attended by relations, friends, co-workers and children from families she had helped with the National Childbirth Trust. The atmosphere was one of cheerful thanksgiving and gratitude to Jane for all she had given and for the wonderful person she was.

An interest in migraine gave me the chance to meet many, both medical and lay, who were outstanding people of achievement, and sometimes I would be asked to give lectures in towns and cities as far away as Glasgow. All this meant that my work was not confined to the area around my general practice. It was also a spur to reading and thinking. There were moments of bizarre comedy. I was once invited to attend a meeting at St. George's Hospital in London on the subject of transcendental meditation: to this day I do not know why I was asked to attend, though I suspect it was because of my interest in relaxation therapy.

We met in the boardroom with portraits in oils of famous medicos glaring sternly down at us. We were to be addressed by the Maharashi Mahash Krishni himself. The press were there in force with floodlights ready for T.V. and video cameras. A sofa had been placed in front of the audience ready for him to sit on crossed legged. It had been covered with a white sheet. Eventually, the Yogi himself appeared, walking forward between the rows of hushed and expectant medicos dressed in the traditional dark suits and ties. He was dressed in white robes and smiled benignly as he seated himself on the white draped sofa.

I cannot remember what he said to us, but I was struck by his theatrical sense and his pleasant humorous personality. After he had spoken there was a discussion on the medical effects of meditation and its effects on the electrical potentials of the brain.

Lecturers who can bring a touch of drama or humour into medical meetings are invaluable as they are remembered when graver and more learned discourses are forgotten. A friend of mine who was a professor of tropical medicine would include in his talks on rabies a demonstration of hydrophobia – a fear of water – with the aid of a full tumbler. His spluttering, coughing and convulsions with water all over the place were not likely to be forgotten by any in his audience.

Lectures on relaxation were apt to be ended with an invitation to the audience to try relaxing for some five minutes or more. Once at a joint talk with members of the dental profession this was so successful that the following lecturer was incensed by the lack of attention by his audience. Stress, tension and anxiety are normal and healthy concomitants of life, but when excessive and unallayed they can cause a temporary breakdown of physiological integration and can occur in migraine, or they can exacerbate other pathological illness.

The understanding and control of damaging stress is an increasingly important aspect of general practice. Once I was asked to see a concert singer having quite severe migraine in the morning of a day when she was due to sing a solo part in a concert with a full orchestra and choir: she had no deputy to take her place. I treated her in ways I have described elsewhere and she recovered enough to avoid cancelling the show. I went to it and sat nervously tense on the edge of my chair until the end and she was acknowledging applause.

Industrial Medicine

My interest in this subject stemmed from my father who was active in the Industrial Welfare Society and who was medical officer for many years to the Army and Navy Stores. As children and adolescents we would be taken to the annual sports day and sometimes I would go with him to boxing matches when he might be greeted by Lord Burghley, the then chairman, and some of the others on the board of managers. He also did sessional work for Carreras cigarettes with their Black Cat label on the packets.

In pre-war days the dangers of smoking had not been realized, and my father himself would smoke a brand of Egyptian cigarettes which most of the family found pungent and disagreeable in regard to the fumes. Now, I feel sure that he might have lived longer if he had not smoked tobacco. In those days it was thought manly to smoke, and an uncle gave me a pipe with tobacco and pouch for a birthday present. Fortunately it gave me nausea when I tried very inexpertly to use it.

During the war my father lived in London with my mother and he continued with his industrial medicine adding to his commitments another factory making highly technical components for the armament industry.

When I went to work at Stourbridge soon after I qualified I made a point of visiting local factories when possible. I would get a cheery greeting when recognised by erstwhile patients and the managements seemed to like us to be shown round. Later on, in the R.A.F., the medical staff were very much implicated in the work of the station and the welfare of the personnel in all sections.

Then, after the war when I was assistant to Dr. Dorothy Campbell, I had the chance to see a bit of the medical problems of the coal-mining industry and some factories doing other work. Once, when visiting a glass factory with doctors doing an industrial course, while watching molten sheets of glass emerging from rollers, an overseas doctor felt ill and had to be taken out. The most interesting section was where lighthouse lanterns were being made and adjusted to high degrees of accuracy.

In general practice I got to know one or two whole time industrial medical officers and some personnel managers, and was able to get a better idea of what various jobs entailed. Then, about 1960, I had the opportunity to do sessional work in a small factory which was part of a major industrial group with units scattered around the British Isles. There was a central medical organization run by a senior industrial medical practitioner with an assistant doctor. They had set up and run a splendid organization which included trained industrial nurses. Every two years there would be a medical meeting for all the doctors and nurses attached as part timers, or in the case of nurses, full timers to the various manufacturing units. We would stay in a pleasant hotel in the country and attend lectures from directors, research people and from doctors with special knowledge of current industrial medical problems.

We would be taken on conducted tours of the various workshops on the site and have the opportunity to talk with the workers, foremen and women, and with departmental managers. They seemed to enjoy telling us about what they did and explaining the different machines and processes.

The world of industry with its hierarchies, ambitions, disappointments, loyalties and stresses is localised and different from those in communities in the outside world, and it had its own medical problems. The rapid changes which can occur in industry in these days give rise to anxieties at all levels, and I have seen management and work practices alter many times in my relatively short connection with industry.

I have witnessed changes ending with a winding down of activities and the recent final closure of the works. This has meant not only anxiety and future uncertainty for many of the employees, some of whom started work in the factory at the age of sixteen and who have given the best part of their working lives to the firm. Their hopes of future employment in a time of recession are poor.

I have been fortunate in being an independent contractor and not subject to the whims and fortunes of a firm in which, as in the services, one has little authority to order one's own life. Those with medical disabilities can be hardest hit, though a deaf and dumb employee I know has now got a post teaching the deaf and dumb language to others. It may not be so easy for a skilled technician with a by-pass graft on his aortic artery to find suitable work and not only will his acquired skills and experience be wasted, but he will lose some of his self confidence and self respect in filling his niche in life.

A visiting doctor from outside the firm like myself could be useful in solving problems facing the unions where health matters were concerned. When a strike was on I would be give a cheery wave by the men on the picket lines as I went in to do my surgery session. On occasions in the past I have acted as go-between for management and shop stewards on disputes with a health element, by having coffee in the surgery with them away from the shop-floor or main offices. In one case a shop steward, thanking me for solving a dispute in which a paranoid worker was making trouble, said 'the man is a bloody nuisance anyway' after being conned into taking this worker's part.

There were occasions of humour too: a charge-hand leaving the workplace to attend a meeting removed his glass eye and placing it on a convenient packing case said to a lazy West African 'remember, I am still keeping my eye on you'. His victim was suitably impressed and went to work with a will.

Language could be a problem with immigrant labour but an appeal to their sense of humour would help to establish a rapport with the West Indians, while some interest in Islamic culture and history would be a help with people from Muslim countries.

Once I had to advise that a heavy-duty lorry driver was suspended from work as he had become subject to what were termed 'dizzy spells'. He challenged this through his union and an important union officer came to the factory ready to make trouble. I gave him and the manager tea in the surgery and we discussed the perils of the road which we were trying to avoid in this case. Eventually, the union man turned to the manager and said 'a medical examination is a bloody good idea; can I have one?' The manager said 'not at the expense of the factory, but ask Dr. Hay'. I saw him privately and at the end he fished out of his pocket a wodge of bank notes saying 'how much is that, doc?'

Stress is something we all have to cope with to a greater or lesser extent, but work can bring a temporary escape from domestic stress, while work stress will affect both efficiency and domestic harmony. Work stress can be particularly threatening to managers who have to appear to be efficient, happy and conforming to the image of a successful and competent manager. A failure to conform can lead to alcoholism, and once when trying to help such a case I found that his chief drinking companion was his general practitioner.

Work on migraine led to me developing an interest in the nature of small muscles areas tender to palpation and the work of Janet Travell and David Simons on the subject. Their detection is a simple matter and can indicate stress from long continued tensing of muscles or they can be initiated by more deep seated disorders of various organs. Having reasonable consultation time in industry, it was possible, with the aid of a competent and interested industrial nurse, to define some problems of stress and sometimes deep seated disorders.

Industrial medical services have done so much to humanize industry in conjunction with the state Employment Medical Service with its accumulated experience. We have come along way since that pioneer of industrial medicine Dr. Charles Turner Thackrah (1795-1833) reported that as many as 50,000 people died annually from the effects of manufacturing. As a student I was never taught much about the perils of industry, though I think that lead poisoning was mentioned as part of the toxicology teaching.

I have enjoyed this part of my professional work and it has broadened my experience in an important side of life and one which should enhance the workers' self respect, but which can do the opposite when arbitrary decisions are made on high which can jeopardise a person's hopes and confidence, such as when closures and redundancies are in the air.

Chapter 10

What It Has All Meant

As has been said the accident of birth decides the environments, cultural and social, in which we find ourselves, and which, even if we try, we cannot deny or wholly discard whatever we may do in later life and wherever we find ourselves.

As a child I grew up in the period following the First World War when the assumptions of the days of Edward the Seventh had gone for ever. Nevertheless, the old ways persisted in my grandmother's house, the social and class distinctions being rigidly preserved and accepted as being the natural order of things sanctified by the Church as we sang 'the rich man in his castle, the poor man at his gate; God made them high and lowly, and ordered their estate'.

Even my mother, the most kindly and considerate of people used the term 'top drawer' to signify the acceptable, or she might break into French if something had to be said of a personal nature within hearing distance of servants who were assumed not to understand the language.

Anglican Church set the seal of respectability. Morning prayer on Sundays complete with sermon was followed by a substantial Sunday lunch.

From an early age we were taken to children's services and sang jolly hymns like Onward Christian Soldiers, and absorbed ideas of gentle Jesus meek and mild pictured with his disciples on stamps which were handed out to us: all were dressed in spotless burnous and wore ascetic, concerned expressions. As part of the Godhead He knew each one of us personally and intimately; even one's inward thoughts and minor misdemeanours were recorded. Forgiveness had to be implored and prayed for.

All this was mystifying and a bit terrifying. We had to recite the catechism and to learn it by heart even if we did not understand it. However, we had fun such as carrying lighted candles in procession: even then I got scolded by Nanny for getting candle grease on my blue serge suit. Handing round the offertory plate, too, was interesting and signified the end of the service with the prospect of lunch followed by a visit to the London zoo. A prod in the ribs which I gave playfully to a schoolfellow as we marched up the aisle side by side to get the takings blessed before the altar, caused him to spill the contents of his plate over the floor losing some coins, mostly pennies and halfpennies with a few farthings, through the gratings covering the hot water pipes.

I do not remember having any very pious feelings at that time and Sunday was rather a day to be endured when one had to be clean and vaguely bored. Sometimes, after church, we would go to Hyde Park to wander among the best people all formally dressed and greeting each other, the men raising their top hats and the elegantly dressed women inclining their heads or offering a hand to be shaken or kissed as they met acquaintances. These Sunday church parades had a charm and elegance now lost in the brasher modern world.

Hyde Park had much to fascinate a child. The tall, handsome lodge keeper at Stanhope Gate dressed in a green uniform complete with a green top hat and a cockade was known to us as Mr. Bottlegreen. Cars in those days came in many exciting shapes and sizes so that traffic watching was fun. There were horses being ridden in Rotten Row, and sometimes one would see the Life Guards looking magnificent on their beautiful horses as they went on their way to Whitehall. These have remained some of my more pleasant and vivid memories of those distant Sundays.

There is no doubt that there is a place for a degree of formality and ritual. Before the last war we were expected to dress for dinner in evening wear, and in a sense this was a compliment to the cook who had prepared the food and to the parlourmaid who served it, and who had prepared the diningroom and set out the table with elegant silverware and table mats. At the time I thought that this was an unnecessary and irksome way of doing things, but now I appreciate its civilizing and cultural value.

At my preparatory school chapel services were better organized and at the evening service when the lights were dimmed for the sermon, I did sometimes get a glimpse of ease and peace in contrast to the usual clamour of school life. We had regular lessons in Old and New Testament and at the end of term were examined on what we were supposed to have learned.

The Old Testament was full of good stories which were interesting if not always edifying by present day standards. The New Testament was accepted, though the ethical teaching did not seem to square with history or some of what we learned about the outside world, but there was always the devil to blame for shortcomings, or the fall of man in Genesis for eating forbidden fruit, a sin which was the cause of much of the world's ills.

Crucifixion was something too horrible to contemplate, and its apparent necessity in the scheme of things eluded me. Even if Christ's physical resurrection was indeed a fact, that hardly concerned the rest of mankind who most assuredly would not be resurrected bodily.

It should be remembered that the slaughter of the First World War was present in the consciousness of the nation from my childhood onwards. However, I was more concerned with coping with day to day problems and the ever present threat of asthmatic attacks. Religion did not bother me until I went to public school. Regular services and house prayers were restful interludes in the more rigorous and unpleasant aspects of life. But, puberty brings with it emotional instability. In my case I revolted inwardly against many of the ideas we were expected to accept uncritically. I learned to keep my feelings to myself, and to adopt as low a profile as was possible.

By the time I got to Cambridge I was agnostic in regard to religion and my brain was occupied enough in studying medicine and passing examinations. But an interest in nature and my experience of something akin to Koestler's 'Oceanic Feeling' at a moment of stress when I was at Château D'Oex remained with me, and it is reassuring to know from the writings of Sir Alistair Hardy and of David Hay (no relation of mine) that others have them.

It has been my good fortune to have had the help and friendship of people I have loved as has already been mentioned, and I have met many fine and courageous people. Some have shown outstanding courage cheerfulness and resources in daunting situations. This was common in war and is commoner than might be thought in seriously ill patients, like the young mother, Jeanette, I have already mentioned.

The tremendous figure of Christ was part of my growing up and one which left me with many uncomfortable questions. Religious and sectarian history gained from school lessons did not square with the life affirming attitudes of much of the New Testament. Church rites and creeds often left me feeling ill at ease even embarrassed.

If Christ, The Life Force, and Life Affirmation are different aspects of the Reality behind the world of the senses, that is a beginning. Christ in his human life was bound to die a physical death for, without death, there could be no evolution in any sense. The fact that in common with many millions of people in history he was killed brutally by the anti-life forces in humanity is part of mankind's story. In that sense much of the Christian tradition is intelligible and it does nothing to exclude the ideas of thoughtful people in other cultures and with other experiences.

All institutions are in danger of reaching a point where their original purposes are obscured by the necessity to expend energy in maintaining their own cohesion; in terms of religion this can mean the formation of exclusive sects prone to decry the experiences of others. This can lead to war, hatred, and fanaticism.

Sir Isaac Newton said 'I do not know what I may appear to the world, but to myself I seem to have been only like a boy playing on the sea-shore, and in diverting myself in now and then finding a smoother pebble or a prettier shell than ordinary, while the great ocean of truth lay all undiscovered before me.'

Our thinking has needed to come to terms with the methods and insights of science and to be conscious of the dangers of the abuse of scientific knowledge at the same time.

There have been moments when the veils of the 'here and now' have appeared to be lifted briefly and these are very personal experiences.

As an outsider who has found little reassurance in sacerdotalism as practised by the churches I have attended, I can appreciate the part played by certain arts and rituals in maintaining social cohesion.

As an example, a great orchestral work means that for a performance a large number of skilled performers have to blend their individualities into a greater whole reflecting the inspiration of the composer. In the background are the instrument makers, the music publishers, the auditorium, the audience and many other items of varying complexity contributing to the production of the whole. This is a useful metaphor for life, but one which can also be applied to life destructive forces.

An Anglican clergyman, a friend from my R.A.F. days, would send up a prayer weekly to the Almighty for the gift of a sense of reality, a sense of proportion, and a sense of humour; a good prescription for those of us who find that life has something in common with a balancing act on a high wire. We fall if reason and feeling are not in some kind of equilibrium.

The ancient myths of the labyrinth express something of our experiences and our fears and reassurances. These are beautifully expressed in a poem of Edwin Muir entitled 'The Labyrinth'. We all need our prophets, teachers, or gurus to make some sense of our experience.

The story of Albert Schweitzer has continued to interest and intrigue me: his regard for personal truth and integrity with his deeply developed ethics of Reverence for Life which led him to leave a successful academic life, to study medicine, and to found a hospital in West Africa make a wonderful story enhancing the meaning and purpose and value in his life. Although pessimistic about the state of the world in his time, he declared himself to be optimistic about the future given more understanding of the ethic he proclaimed.

Any inherited disability, including asthma, tends to make one turn in on oneself and to hide one's problem from other people as far as possible with the ever present fear of failure. Nevertheless, each difficulty overcome is a boost to self confidence which can bring many rewards. Mine have come from the privilege of being in the medical profession dealing with individual persons and from an interest in nature, the sea and the country. For all these I am deeply grateful.